Techniques for Health & Wholeness

OTHER BOOKS BY BETTY BETHARDS:

Atlantis
Be Your Own Guru
The Dream Book
Relationships in the New Age of Aids
Sex & Psychic Energy
There is No Death
Way To Awareness

Cassette tapes also available. For free newsletter, Send S.A.S.E. to:

Inner Light Foundation
P.O. Box 750265
Petaluma, CA 94975

Techniques for Health & Wholeness

Healing of Body, Mind and Spirit

Betty Bethards

Inner Light Foundation Petaluma California

The Inner Light Foundation is a non-profit, non-denominational organization engaged in teaching, healing, research and publishing. Formed in 1969, the ILF extends its basic meditation teaching to self-help techniques in the areas of interpersonal communication, health/wellness, emotional and spiritual growth.
Activities of the ILF include monthly lectures, weekend seminars, and media appearances.

Betty Bethards is the founder of the ILF

First Printing: November 1980
Second Printing: September 1983
Third Printing: July 1985
Fourth Printing: April 1991
Fifth Printing: May 1992

Book Design: Jon Goodchild
Cover illustration: John Newman
Photography: Wernher Krutein

Printed in the United States of America

ISBN: 0-918915-17-1

This book is lovingly
dedicated to my children,
Pam, and Dave, without whose love,
encouragement and support it would not
have been possible.

Contents

Preface 11

Chapter 1: Introduction to Health and Wholeness 13

Everyone Can Heal Wholistic Health What Is Health? Causes of Disease What About Accidents? Reincarnation, An Expanded View Karma and Death Using Your Healing Power

Chapter 2: Understanding the Healing Energy 25

You Are an Energy Being Energy and the Chakras The Root Chakra The Second Chakra The Third Chakra The Heart Center The Fifth Chakra The Sixth Chakra The Crown Chakra Energy and the Male-Female Polarities High Energy and a Good Attitude Healing Energy and Cycles High Energy, Health and Meditation

Chapter 3: The Nature of Disease 39

It's All in Your Mind Understanding Fear Facing What You Fear Buttons and Programs Aging, A Negative Program Emotional Trauma and Mental Illness Playing the Game Too Wide Open The Psychics Possession Disease, an Imbalance

Chapter 4: Healing Yourself 55

You Deserve Health The Most Effective Tools Relaxation Meditation Affirmation Visualization Relaxation Techniques The Inner Light Foundation Meditation Technique Affirmations for Health Visualization Techniques Self-Healing Through Dreams Natural Methods for Self-Healing

Chapter 5: Sending Healing to Others 81

Healing Is an Inside Job Your Role in Sending Healing Energy When Healing Doesn't Work Can Everyone Heal? The Basic Healing Group Etheric Surgery Clearing the Chakras Finding Energy Blocks in the Spine Third Eye Combing the Aura Fluffing the Aura Foot Massage Absent Healing Natural Group Healing

Chapter 6: Healing the World Through Spiritual Awareness 101

Love Is the Secret Seeing the God-Self The Second Coming The Guru Lies Within A Basic Lesson in Unity An Exercise in Awareness The Importance of Learning to Heal

Preface

Betty Bethards is widely known as a spiritual healer, meditation teacher, psychic and mystic. She has been called a superwoman of the supernatural and one of the top psychic healers in this country.

Betty was taught methods of healing and meditation by her *channel.* Her channel, she explains, is her attunement to her inner guides and teachers. What she channels comes *through* her, from higher sources of wisdom and insight. It is the intuitional level of awareness, a high frequency or rate of vibration that one learns to hear by attuning to finer energies within. Everyone has a channel, she believes, and can open to the insight and love energy that comes from these expanded levels of consciousness.

Over the last twelve years Betty has been spreading the teachings of her channel to thousands of people. These and other healing techniques are included in this volume.

"Physician, heal thyself," is her basic message in *Techniques for Health and Wholeness.* The Physician within you is your higher self, or God-self, and knows all answers to your problems of health and everyday living. As we learn to get in touch with this inner self, and accept responsibility for our own health and well-being, a whole new world of harmony and happiness opens to each one of us.

Chapter 1

Introduction to Health and Wholeness

Everyone Can Heal

Each one of us has healing power. We can heal ourselves, our relationships, and our environment. We can help others learn how to use their healing ability, and all work together to create a world of harmony and wholeness.

This was one of the most exciting truths revealed to me when I first began meditating and developing my psychic abilities. Whenever I would get discouraged with my progress in meditation, the promise of learning to heal always kept me going. Even today healing is my first love, because it means bringing the whole man into perfect balance and awakening the true God nature within.

Today spiritual healing is enjoying a new wave of interest and popularity. Healing groups of caring individuals meet regularly throughout the world to serve as pillars of healing energy and love for others to draw upon. Alternative methods of healing, including spiritual healing, are taught in some nursing schools and discussed at medical conferences. Well-known healers are asked to assist medical professionals with some of their patients. But no matter who the healer or what the method, all healing comes from God, or the God-self within.

All healing, in fact, is Self-healing. The doctor can dress the wound, the healer can send energy, but it is the Physician within who restores health. We ourselves must accept responsibility for our health.

Wholistic Health

The wholistic health movement is gaining momentum today, and among other things emphasizes individual responsibility. It includes all of the healing arts, draws from both eastern and western traditions, and addresses itself to the total man: physical, mental and spiritual. Traditional medicine, acupuncture, reflexology, psychic and spiritual healing, meditation, massage, herbology, color therapy, psychotheraphy, biofeedback and many other areas are included within its scope.

As its name suggests, wholistic health seeks to treat the *whole* man. We simply cannot treat the symptom alone without getting at the cause, or the disease will manifest somewhere else in a different form. It is time to integrate our awareness of ourselves as physical, mental and spiritual beings. It is time to integrate our knowledge from all areas, all traditions, to be open to both the old and the new, to learn as much as we can from every phase and form of healing.

Traditionally medical science has tended to brand all unorthodox methods of healing that produced results as faith healing. These methods work, it said, because the disease is psychosomatic, and because of the placebo effect, or the belief in the patient's own mind that he is being helped.

There is truth in this, of course, but in fact *every* illness and *every* condition of disease we bring upon ourselves through our own thoughts. Ultimately it is our own attitudes, our own choices, that create our life experiences.

What Is Health?

My channel has explained that "a healthy person is one who is balanced emotionally, physically and spiritually, and one who has balanced the masculine and feminine energies within. A healthy person is one who can love himself, who can take time to play, to rest, to create, to give and receive. But most of all if one is healthy he is following his own destiny, fulfilling his own potentials, and manifesting personal happiness and vitality in every area of his life."

Health represents a dynamic state of balance, or equilibrium. Our health at any given moment reflects our mental, emotional, physical and spiritual state of understanding. Health means being fulfilled and balanced in every area of our lives: personal, social, financial, professional. Our lack of well-being in any given area is the result of our negative thinking or mental programs, and no one else is to blame.

Causes of Disease

Disease may be caused by negativity or unenlightened beliefs about ourselves and the nature of God.

Negativity takes many forms, but always has its worst effect on the person thinking negatively. Stemming from fear, it may be experienced as guilt, hatred, envy, insecurity, or numerous other things. These thoughts held in the mind produce disastrous results in the body.

Also, a major limiting belief about the nature of God can invite disharmony into our lives. Perhaps your understanding of the Divine Being does not include a picture of a God of love and harmony, or your notion of God is overshadowed by the Judge and Punisher (I use the term *God* because I am comfortable with it, but you may substitute anything you wish: Cosmic Intelligence, Divine Love, Universal Mind, Life Principle, or whatever.)

Many of us have been programmed to believe that poor health is in some way a virtue, or that each of us must have a cross to bear if we would be holy. But that is from the old hellfire and damnation tradition that suggests that to suffer for the Lord is good, and that God tries those He loves. (I know that line very well, having grown up in a fundamentalist Baptist group. I learned to *fear* God, and never knew about the God of love and joy until I was much older.) So we may subconsciously welcome hardship and sickness as a way of making us special, or think this is more morally acceptable than being happy and having all the things in life we want.

But God is not a judge and punisher, perched on a throne doling out little hardships to test us. That view, in fact, is a tremendous cop-out for accepting responsibility for what is happening in our lives.

Our natural state of being is harmony. If we are experiencing disharmony in any area of living, it is because we are not attuning to the infinite spirit within us and beginning to recognize the limiting belief or attitude that has brought on the condition.

What About Accidents?

If all disease begins and ends in the mind, you may be asking, what about things like car accidents, or plane crashes where everyone is killed? Surely people don't create disasters!

Here let me state emphatically that there is no such thing as coincidence, and nothing happens by chance! There is a lesson and meaning behind everything in our lives, and we in some way have contributed to its manifestation.

For example, if a man has been physically active all his life and is in a car accident and breaks his leg, it can be a blessing in disguise. Perhaps he needed to slow down or he would have had a heart attack. Or, by having a close brush with death and suddenly being grounded, he may find it is a time of intensive self-therapy, examining and redirecting his life goals. (It doesn't mean we have to take such drastic measures, but some of us are so stubborn that it takes a lot to get our attention!)

If one crosses over in a plane crash it represents having good karma, because that is an easy and effortless way to leave the earth plane. And you can be sure if it wasn't someone's time to go, he wouldn't be on the plane in the first place.

Reincarnation, an Expanded View

But there is another consideration: why are some people born blind, deaf, or with some other debilitating condition? As a child I always wondered why life seemed so unfair, and not until I began to accept the idea of reincarnation, taught me by my inner guides and teachers, did things begin to make a little more sense. (Whether you believe in reincarnation is not that important. I resisted it for a long time, coming from a fundamentalist background. You should always take what feels right to you and chuck the rest. We each have our own truths, and your soul knows what is truth for you.)

In a nutshell, reincarnation is the idea that we have so much to learn here on the earth plane that we couldn't possibly do it in just one lifetime. So we keep coming back, incarnating again and again, until we have achieved that perfect physical, mental and spiritual balance we all are striving for (whether we consciously know it or not).

And each time we choose our circumstances and conditions very carefully. We choose our race, sex, parents, place and date of birth, and economic conditions. And we carefully choose the kind of body we want, the physical vehicle we think will help us grow and learn the most. We are never born into anything less than a perfect body unless we choose it. For example, if a person wants to be forced to develop his inner perception, psychic or clairvoyant ability, he may choose to be born blind.

My channel has explained:

The earth plane and what you term disease is here merely as a teacher. Many people will choose to undergo physical disabilities in an incarnation, but only as a positive thing forcing them to develop their other potentials. When man has excellent health at all times he often abuses it and fails to develop deeper creative potential which calls for more disciplined effort and self-examination. Many situations you see as unfair: people who are crippled, mentally retarded, or sense impaired. But these souls are working on other gifts. They have deliberately chosen to place an obstacle before themselves so that they will manifest their highest potential in other areas.

Sometimes a soul will deliberately choose to be physically ugly or marred on some way to learn to manifest beauty from within. The external part of man is only a shell, mask, or the suit of clothes he has chosen to wear. This is an important lesson to learn. And when the external vehicle is damaged in any way man must often stop and review his life, asking, "What am I doing? What is my purpose? Am I the body of something much more?"

Reincarnation places the responsibility solely on the individual. As you sow you reap. As you choose, you experience. There is no room to blame your parents, your spouse, your children, or any other aspect of your situation for causing your poor health. When you incarnate you know where you have weaknesses and where you have strengths. Experiences are simply teaching you various lessons.

If you are asking why you would choose to incarnate in a seemingly negative environment, it is probably because you generated the same negative behavior to others in a previous lifetime and you want to learn why not to do it. But remember you are always a free agent, and may choose to respond to anything in a positive or negative way. It is your own attitude, even as a child, that determines your reality. For example, if your parents are alcoholics, you can use their behavior as an excuse to feel sorry for yourself or you may use it as an opportunity to recognize how they are setting up their lives and choose not to make the same mistake.

Everything is your own choice, whether in this life, another life, or between lives. But whatever you have chosen, you can begin to develop balance within, learning to manifest more and more each day total health and well-being. The blind can be cured, the lame can learn to walk. Ultimately, there is no condition too great or too small to be healed once we have learned the lesson it had to teach us. My channel has said that some day we will be able to correct virtually all conditions; we will even learn how to grow new limbs and organs.

Each one of us can contribute to this advancing understanding of energy through exploring and working on our own conditions of imbalance. At that time of advanced knowledge it will be clearly seen how thought is the molder of health and disease. The technology will be there to correct many conditions; man's thinking must maintain the desired state of health.

Karma and Death

When you are suffering from a particular condition, you should not adopt an attitude of resignation, saying, "I guess I'll always have such and such. That's my karma. I created it and will have to live with it." Learn the lesson from the disease and transcend it! (Techniques for insight into the cause of disharmony are given in Chapter 4).

When another person is experiencing disease or disharmony, it is never for you to say, "Oh, I can't help you. That's your karma." Nor should we concern ourselves with whether we should send healing energy to one who has been labeled terminally ill. Your extra energy and love can be the positive boost someone needs to get insight into the nature of his condition and overcome it. Sending energy to the terminally ill person will either help restore him to health or provide extra energy to cross over if it is time for his transition. Energy at "death" is as important as energy and support at birth.

We should not think of death as the antithesis to health. Life and death are really two sides of the same coin. They are simply fluctuations, waves, in the cosmic energy of God. Death is simply leaving the body, and we all leave the body at night anyway when we dream. At physical death we simply go out and don't return.

What we call life on earth is really a school, and those who have died are much more alive than we are.

Life here is a lot of work. We have many lessons to learn. When it is time for us to leave the earth plane, shed our physical body and change our rate of vibration, we have truly earned it. I call it earning your R and R (rest and recuperation)!

You may ask, "Are painful deaths necessary? Why do so many seem to linger in suffering?" Often when a person chooses a slow or painful departure it is because he has never learned to receive from others. In this way he is forced to depend upon the love and good will of others to aid him. But once a lesson is recognized in a situation, there is no reason for the pain to continue.

This has been true of many cancer patients, for example. Those dying of cancer, realizing the meaning of their life and getting in touch with the lessons of the disease, have suddenly found that all the pain is gone. If it is their time to cross over, they will then have a beautiful and peaceful transition. If it is not, they will begin to "miraculously" recover and the disharmony will completely leave their system as new patterns of thought and insight take over.

We should look at all diseases and experiences along the way as opportunities for learning, explore them, and move beyond them. We will all leave the earth plane, but we do not have to go through the transition in sickness and pain. Death should be a beautiful new birth experience into an expanded realm of consciousness, and we can be fully aware and experiencing every moment as an exhilerating journey.

Realizing death is a natural process, however, does not give us the license to commit suicide. We are given a body to help us work through our problems. At death you are still faced with the same lessons if you haven't learned them on the earth plane. A suicide will cost you from six to eight incarnations, and you will have to meet the same circumstances again and be able to walk through them in a future life. So you might as well hang in and learn all you can!

Using Your Healing Power

No matter what your age or condition, your background or interests, you can begin to use your healing power immediately. You don't even have to believe in it, but a little belief goes a long way.

When I first began working with a healing group, practicing the techniques that my inner teachers were giving me, I was very skeptical and so were the group members. But they worked in spite of us. As soon as I began to realize, "Hey, this stuff really works!" I was hooked for life. Through the years I have worked with persons who have recovered from terminal illnesses, brain tumors, cancer, ulcers, and all manner of diseases. I have come to realize that what we call miraculous is simply the result of learning to use and understand our God given abilities. I have seen how healing techniques and meditation can restore health, and I have also seen how disease can return again if meditation and the new orientation toward oneself and others is not maintained.

The whole purpose of this book is to enable you to awaken your healing potential, and to learn to act independently — to follow your own intuition — in accepting responsibility for your health and well-being.

A number of techniques are given in Chapters 4 and 5, which combine many methods including etheric surgery and directing energy through the chakras which I was taught by my channel. Practice them, work with them, then develop your own style. There is no right or wrong way to send healing. It can be done through touching or not touching, in someone's presence or from thousands of miles away. For sending healing is really just sending love.

If we are to maintain a new state of health and harmony, we must realize that all true healing is spiritual healing, because through love we transform the deepest levels within our beings.

These techniques are not suggested to be used instead of traditional medical treatment, but to work hand in hand with the best methods available from all traditions.

Chapter 2

Understanding the Healing Energy

You Are an Energy Being

It is easy to understand healing if you think of yourself as an electrical system. We are energy beings, systems of interpenetrating energy fields. What we perceive as the physical body is only one level of vibration within the total system.

Our teachers on the other side, and those persons who perceive clairvoyantly, don't see us as solid at all. They see us as levels of vibration within an energy field. They see how smoothly the energy is flowing, whether it is blocked, and how much we can hold and process within our systems. This determines our state of physical, mental and spiritual health.

The body as vibration is fluid and pliable. It can easily be molded into a state of health or a state of disease, depending upon our thinking. Our thoughts move easily throughout the body, and every cell is alive with intelligence. We are constantly building up or tearing down by our behavior patterns and thinking habits. So we are always in the process of creating harmony or disharmony within. We must catch on to this idea that we are *dynamic life energy* if we would truly understand the healing process.

The energy that surrounds and interpenetrates the physical body is called the etheric body, or aura. A lot of scientific research has been done on the aura in recent years. Efforts have been made through Kirlian photography to photograph the energy emanating from the body. But current research has hardly scratched the surface, and has not been able to record the true etheric body or spiritual energy of the individual.

But what is this energy? It is the life force, the healing energy, kundalini, prana, holy spirit, or whatever you want to call it. The ancient Hawaiians called it mana, the Chinese knew it as ch'i, and it has been known in almost every ancient tradition. It permeates all life, it *IS* life, and fills the universe. It is the essence of our beings. It is the God energy, or love energy. Call it what you will, but how you use and process it determines how you experience reality.

Energy and the Chakras

We in the western world have only recently begun to understand that man is an intricate energy system. This knowledge was built into Chinese medicine in the practice of acupuncture thousands of years ago, and today is finding its way into western medicine. Knowledge of this energy has also been the basis of the martial arts, the true masters understanding the power and flow of these forces within man's being.

Also, thousands of years ago the Hindu tradition recognized seven major energy centers within man. These were called *chakras,* a Sanskrit word meaning wheel, because clairvoyants who could see these centers described them as spinning wheels of energy.

The chakras are like transformers, joining the etheric body with the physical, and they step down the rate of vibration so that it can be handled in the physical system. They correspond roughly as the etheric dimension of the endocrine glands, and are located at the base of the spine, in the sexual organs, the solar plexus, heart, throat, between the eyebrows, and the crown of the head. (Although I have discussed these in some detail in my book *Sex and Psychic Energy,* I will elaborate again here because they are crucial to understanding healing.)

Each chakra represents a way of understanding ourselves and the world, a way of perceiving reality. If we suppress or block energy at any of these levels, disease will manifest in the corresponding area of the body. Different diseases will manifest as a result of blockage in any given chakra depending upon an individual's mental and physical makeup. Also, if a chakra is too wide open disease may result, for we would not have control over the amount of energy flowing through it.

Our health depends upon a dynamic balance of energy among all the chakras, plus a balance of the male and female polarities within. We must learn how to awaken and direct energy through our systems to maintain maximum health and well-being.

It is important to realize that all of the chakras are open to a degree, but we tend to operate out of some more than others. In each individual one or two will be weaker than the rest, and it is in the weak or blocked ones that tension or disease will manifest. Emotional suppression, for example, will manifest as disease in the area where there is the least energy — a blocked chakra — and then can spread to other areas. Cancer, a result of suppression, manifests behind whatever chakra is blocked. This can be a result of tension, fear, negative thinking, or sitting on your own unhappiness and not making changes. It is the end result of your lack of awareness. The key is to open the system, cleanse and flush out the energy field with the natural healing processes, and release the negative thought patterns that are responsible for the disharmony in the first place.

The Root Chakra

The healing energy or kundalini (and I prefer to call it kundalini because it's the term my channel gave me) is housed at the base of the spine. The first or root chakra serves as a trigger to release this energy. When a healer is working with someone, what he is really doing is getting the patient's kundalini flowing up and down the spine. In this way the patient's own energy is awakening and balancing the chakras, beginning the healing process.

In the first chakra there would be no energy blocks. The first is like a storage bank for the kundalini. The kundalini comes up naturally twice in our lives, once at puberty and again at menapause. At puberty when the kundalini is activated it is bringing the entity into the awareness that he or she is a particular physical vibration, and the male and female chemistry comes into alignment. In addition to the heightened sexual awareness, however, it is also a time of creativity.

Again at menapause, which both men and women experience, the kundalini kicks up as another chance to use this life energy to renew your physical, mental and spiritual being. A hormonal change is involved for both men and women. The energy often gets stuck in the second or sexual chakra, and people choose to have what they call one last fling before settling into old age. But if the energy was truly understood it could be transmuted into a higher level of vigor and well-being. It certainly should not signify that one is going over the hill, but rather that he now has a heightened creativity which can propel him to great productivity and fulfillment.

These times of puberty and menapause are stressful due to the changes taking place, but through an understanding of energy and the practice of meditation they can be heightened periods of growth which open the door to continued vitality.

But ideally we learn to trigger this energy from the root chakra whenever it is needed, to use it to maintain a high level of awareness at all times. The important thing to remember here is that it is always with you as an infinite reservoir of vitality and strength.

The Second Chakra

The second or sexual chakra is the first that can be blocked. Suppression of energy here may result from fears and guilts about sex, feeling inadequate in one's sexual role, having sex infrequently, being in a bad marriage, feeling unfulfilled in love and sleeping around, holding on to unpleasant memories from previous relationships, or trying to lead a celibate life and not understanding how to channel the energy into higher centers.

The suppression is expressed as violence, explosions of anger, prostate or female organ problems, colitis, and other physical ailments in the lower abdominal region.

It is important to utilize and release the energy in the second chakra in some way, whether through masturbation, a creative outlet, sexual intercourse, meditation, or a combination of these. It is vital that we get in touch with our sexual needs and determine whether we are blocking energy in this center.

The Third Chakra

The third chakra or solar plexus is the area in which most people experience their difficulties, particularly sensitive people. This is what I call the worry chakra. It is a very vulnerable center.

If this chakra isn't balanced or is too wide open, a person will pick up everyone else's trips, whether positive or negative. One will experience extreme nervousness, be high strung, and may find himself with ulcers, gall bladder problems, or cancer of the stomach.

To balance this chakra one needs to learn how to detach from other people's trips, which is best done through building the energy in meditation, getting more physical exercise, and using the energy in some creative outlet. When this center is balanced it can serve as a valuable intuitive guide, for then it is no longer swayed by fear and anxiety.

The Heart Center

The heart center or fourth chakra is the first of the higher creative centers. This is the center of the Christ spirit, or unconditional love for oneself and one's fellows. It is a beautiful level through which one experiences unity with all life. But it has a dual problem.

First, if it is too wide open you will pick up all the suffering and the pain of the human condition, being unable to detach and gain a perspective on it.

This has always been one of my biggest problems: I'll be so aware of your hurting that I'll be out there trying to clear it up for you, rather than seeing how you set it up and what you are learning from it. This leads to playing the mother-counselor or father-counselor role, which is very safe. It is all right to play that some of the time, but we also need to work with someone in a one to one relationship in which we become vulnerable enough to look at our own numbers.

Second, if the heart center is closed or walled off, you will be unable to love yourself and others. Being walled off in this center not only blocks you from being sensitive to another's feelings, but will result in high blood pressure and heart problems. (We build up and carry around many resentments and hurts here, overloading this area with unnecessary tension.)

The ideal is to be open and channeling energy from this center, but perceiving from a more objective chakra, such as the third eye or crown.

The Fifth Chakra

The fifth center is associated with higher creativity and clairaudience (psychic hearing or perception of finer vibrations), and it is easy to block through tension. Blocks here manifest most readily as tension in the back of the neck, often resulting in backaches, headaches and eyestrain. Throat problems also result from suppression in the fifth center.

Other blocks are caused through lack of verbalization of one's real needs and feelings. Expressing your creative ability, communication with yourself and others, are important to the proper functioning of this center.

The Sixth Chakra

The sixth center, also known as the third eye, is not a contributor to much illness. If a person has been concentrating for long hours he may experience a buildup of tension between the eyes, resulting in sinus headache or eyestrain, although usually this is a result of blockage in the fifth. The third eye merges into the crown or seventh chakra after a person has been meditating for awhile, and the two are as one center.

The third eye is associated with the opening of true psychic potential and spiritual knowledge, seeing with the one eye of truth. When one has learned to direct energy through this center it can be a powerful healing beam, stronger than a laser.

The Crown Chakra

You never find any disease coming from the crown center. This represents union with the God self. Pictures of saints and religious teachers often show a ring of light around the head, seen by poets, artists and clairvoyants, which is the emanation of energy from the merger of the sixth and seventh chakras.

Energy and the Male-Female Polarities

Earlier I mentioned that we are trying to learn to balance the male and female energies of our being in addition to opening up and balancing the chakras. The male-female polarity in the body is associated with the concepts of yin-yang, creative-receptive, the positive and negative, the intellect and intuition. Each one of us is both male and female, manifesting in a particular body.

These aspects are also associated with the right and left sides of the brain. The right represents intuition, creativity and higher awareness, and the left represents reason, intellect, time and linear awareness. The left helps us stay grounded and function in the space-time world, but for the most part it has been greatly overemphasized and we have begun to see it as the only reality. The right side is our door to God consciousness; it is the feeling, intuiting side. It is the dimension that can give us all the answers to our daily problems, correct any imbalance in our health, because it puts us in touch with the Physician within. We need both the right and the left, but they must work together in an dynamic blending and balance.

The male and female roles in society are conditioned at an early age, although this is beginning to change with the advent of women's liberation, gay liberation, and other equal rights movements. Typically men aren't supposed to feel, to cry, or to be in touch with their deeper sensitivity. This is why so often men put up their walls, especially when going through puberty, and block a lot of their creativity. Men die earlier than women, suffer from more heart attacks and other stress related diseases because of this suppression of energy.

Women have not been taught to suppress this feeling side, and it is more acceptable for them to cry, vent their emotions, and express affection. The feeling, intuiting side is thus more developed. "A woman's intuition" is an acceptable way of knowing for females.

But men should be as intuitive as women, and women should be as rational as men, because we are a combination of these energies. We will choose a woman's body if we are working on developing our sensitivity, and a man's if we are trying to bring through more strengths. So the idea of liberating ourselves from set roles is an important step in beginning to realize the duality of our natures.

Homosexuality is nothing more than a time of transition from a male to a female body, or vice versa. If you were a woman in your last life and suddenly find yourself in a man's body, you may still feel like a woman. There is nothing wrong with having particular sexual preferences, but the important thing is that you learn whatever lessons you came back to learn, and not get caught up in focusing all your energy in the second chakra. We have all been homosexuals in one lifetime or another, and this should be viewed as simply a time of balancing energies and growing in self-awareness as in any other lifetime.

High Energy and a Good Attitude

I have said that how high your energy is determines your state of health. Energy is, in addition, the key to understanding your attitudes and behavior.

The effects of a changing energy level can be seen quite easily in the rapid changes of mood that many people experience. You suddenly feel depressed. You look around for all kinds of reasons, analyze things, but the basic cause of depression is that your energy has dropped. If your energy was high, then whatever just happened to bother you or get you down would have rolled right off your back.

Energy can drop because you are too wide open and pick up someone else's trip, because you yourself are thinking negatively or worrying, because you've been working or studying a long time and your body is tense. If we stay locked in the intellect for a long time we get out of balance and lose our energy. (Remember it is the creative energy that restores and rejuvenates you.)

When this happens, rather than getting mad at everyone around you, you can learn to stop and reflect: Okay, my energy just dropped on me. What have I been doing? Did I forget to eat? Relax? Take time to play? Am I worrying too much? What am I doing wrong? Did I forget to close down and pick up someone else's trip? It is at this point that we need to stop and do something creative, get outside, take a short trip, meditate, or whatever. Don't stay indoors, pull the drapes, and feel sorry for yourself.

Also, watching television for too long is a major energy rip off, and a lot of kids are experiencing suicidal tendencies at an age when they should be full of vigor and enthusiasm for life. They aren't using their energy, and it is being drained into the tube, and they wonder why they get depressed.

All of us have these regenerative forces within us, but we must remember to use them.

Healing Energy and Cycles

Every seven years we go through health cycles, just as we go through seven year cycles in relationships, jobs, chronological age, and so on. Every seven years every cell in your body has been replaced, and your psychological attitude has changed.

If we are aware of the various cycles we are in at any given time — job, age, relationships — then we can be more prepared when we approach the transition periods. The seventh year of any cycle can be a time of additional stress if we do not understand what is happening. But if we are meditating we can watch things in a detached way, knowing that the old is passing and the new is moving into our experience.

My channel has said that it takes seven years for a disease to manifest in the physical body from the time it begins in one's thought patterns. For example, if you discover you have cancer or stomach ulcers, the source of the problem would have begun seven years earlier. It may appear to have come on suddenly, but in fact has been building in your energy field for a long time. (This does not hold true for minor imbalances or for colds and viruses, which are cleansing agents.)

And this is important to realize. Disease manifests in the energy field before it manifests in the physical body. This is why one can look at the aura and tell whether a person is going to be sick, even when the person is showing no signs of approaching illness. Of course, as you become more sensitive to energy through meditation you will become aware of your extended energy body, and can detect and correct subtle changes as they arise.

You have heard that prevention is the best cure. We should become so sensitive to the balance of energy within us that we can eliminate all tension and negativity causing energy blocks before it ever has a chance to manifest as physical illness.

High Energy, Health and Meditation

What we call resistance to disease is also a result of high energy. If the body is imbalanced, in a run down state, one will be more likely to pick up whatever is in the air. Negative attitudes, depression, boredom and confusion dissipate the body's energy and leave you wide open.

But if your psychological attitude is positive, your energy high, then chances are that everyone in your family could get a particular disease and it would not affect you at all.

The easiest way to keep your energy high and cleanse the chakras is through daily meditation. In the meditation process you are relaxing and bringing up the kundalini to heal and harmonize the energy systems of your body.

Meditation is really the key to building your own energy field, your resistance to disease, because every time you meditate you are recharging your batteries. Each and every cell in the body contains interdimensional atoms of energy, and if you're meditating you are revitalizing every cell and energy level in the physical and etheric bodies. You are keeping them light, and raising your overall level of awareness. Negativity and blocks will be dislodged from your system, because they are weights that cannot stay within an en-lightened body. They will come up and out, and the hurts you have suppressed will have to be looked at and let go.

The self and group healing techniques given in Chapters 4 and 5 are most effective when used hand in hand with meditation. No matter how simple these processes appear, they all involve awakening the system to its natural healing processes. Remember you can learn to channel energy through your system, let go of blocks, negative thinking and disease at any age.

Chapter 3

The Nature of Disease

It's All in Your Mind

The real cause of disease begins and ends in your mind. All disharmony, discomfort and imbalance are self-inflicted.

Today we hear a lot about psychosomatic illness, which merely suggests that a belief, stress or mental hang-up is the creator of a physical condition. More and more doctors are beginning to believe that a high percentage of all illness does stem from stress: allergies, ulcers, cancer, diabetes, constipation, just to name a few.

This stress is a block in the system, or can be the result of a chakra being too wide open and depleting one of energy. Stress changes the whole chemical make-up of the physical body, and alters the functioning of the endocrine glands and energy centers.

A certain amount of stress or tone in the muscles and organs is essential, maintaining a dynamic balance and healthy functioning. But our self-imposed stresses, built up over a long period of time, are debilitating. Stress can be a good friend, helping us to look at our fears and negative responses, but it can also be an enemy when unheeded.

We must learn to release physical and mental stress at the end of each day so we do not keep building up tension and suppressing feelings.

The root emotion behind stress, behind disease, is fear. Fear manifests in a thousand ways, as hatred, envy, guilt, jealousy, greed, hurt, and all the other negative emotions you could name. Fear in its many guises is most responsible for creating stress within the system.

Understanding Fear

The fear of rejection is probably man's biggest fear, but he also has the fear of living, the fear of dying, the fear of loving, the fear of being unloved, unwanted, uncared for, the fear of failure, the fear of success, and the fear of responsibility. This is what sets the mental programs in motion that affect his health and drains so much of his energy.

Fear grows within us when we do not love ourselves. Genuine self-love recognizes the God within, the radiant being who is growing and learning and has the answer to every problem. Lack of self-love is the greatest cause of destruction within the physical, mental and spiritual being. If you do not love yourself, you cannot let anyone else love you, and you can't love others. You'll always feel inferior to other people, comparing yourself and feeling insecure around them.

Life is not supposed to be a competitive game, but should merely provide a growing and acceleration point for each and every soul. Some are working on developing the intellect because they had no interest in this in past lives, some are working on developing their creative aspects, some are working on developing a beginning spiritual awareness. But each one is working on something that is just as important to him as the next. And one must really love the self within to understand what his major task is for this lifetime, and in turn not be so concerned with how others choose to lead their lives.

If we could really learn this self-love, my channel has often emphasized, honoring our own growth and the growth of our fellows, we would be free from all illness and stress related problems.

Our guilts are also a result of fear, not living up to expectations, afraid of looking bad in the eyes of others. Guilts stem from fear of criticism and authoritarian figures, fear of daring to be ourselves, fear of change. People will stay in a relationship or job situation when the body is telling them that it will literally kill them with stress if they don't leave.

Recently my channel called fear the last fortress. It is the last stronghold we cling to that separates us from our true selves. We build walls around ourselves, fortifying ourselves, against what? All those imagined threats and terrors we create within our own minds.

We must learn there is nothing to fear but our own negativity, begin looking at and overcoming our fears one by one, and opening the doors to our fear fortress. Then we can tear down all the walls and allow the love force to flow into every corner of our beings.

This is true on a personal, national and international scale: we must become aware of our unity and overcome the fear consciousness that has separated us for so long from one another.

Facing What You Fear

We must learn to look at each and every fear, to meet whatever we are afraid of. There is an old truism: You must face what you fear. This has a double meaning.

First, if you are afraid of something you hold it in your mind, and you will attract it to yourself. In the laws of mind, like attracts like. If you're afraid of being robbed, you'll put the vibration out there and someone will come in and do you the favor. If you are afraid you can't trust people, they won't disappoint you because you are setting it up. If you are afraid of being rejected—which has always been one of my big ones—you will attract situations to yourself again and again in which you can play out your rejection number, until finally you learn you are worthy of love and bring that into your life instead.

So, on the one hand, we must face what we fear because we will draw it to us simply by dwelling upon it. The second meaning concerns overcoming the problem. For as soon as we turn around and face the thing we have been running from, it no longer has any power over us. As soon as we are able to say, "Hey, this is a fear I have, let's see where it is coming from and how I can let it go," it will begin to effortlessly vanish.

For example, let's say I am afraid of failing in my business. Many men fear this one. We have to look at that fear, asking ourselves: "What's the worst thing that could possibly happen?" Obviously, that we could lose everything. But the mind is unlimited, and what we once create we can create again. History is full of stories about millionaires who made a fortune, lost every penny of it, then created an even bigger one. There are people who lose it all and go into the depths of depression, and those who lose it all and realize that the outer things are merely symbols of inner resources, that each one of us has an unlimited supply.

There is really no way in life to fail. We make mistakes in order to learn. There is no such thing as blowing the perfect opportunity. If you aren't ready for something, or you run a negative number and blow a relationship or job opportunity, fine. See what you did, how you set it up, learn from it, and create an even better situation for yourself. But if you don't realize that you set up a negative situation and try to blame everyone else, you will continually draw disappointments to yourself, creating the same scene over and over again.

Buttons and Programs

I often talk about getting your buttons pushed and running your programs in my lectures, and sometimes I am asked just what I mean.

A button is a vulnerable spot, a fear spot within your mind. It comes out of some experience or belief in which you feel threatened. A button represents an addiction to a negative emotion.

For example, if you are very sensitive about your appearance (you fear rejection if you don't look a certain way) and someone makes a snide remark about something you're wearing, you'll get your button pushed. You'll probably become emotionally uptight and feel embarrassed, get defensive. All you really have to do is smile and say, "Too bad. I like it."

Or, one of my favorites used to be if my husband walked off without telling me where he was going I immediately thought I'd done something wrong (a basic insecurity).

Anything you react to, become upset by, anything that causes an unsettling emotional reaction represents a button.

A program is a belief about yourself, and is the foundation for buttons. If you believe you are unworthy, unattractive, unskilled, or whatever, you will have correspondingly appropriate buttons.

Programs and buttons are always tied up with our past experiences, whether in this life or a past life. Most of us refer to our past to describe ourselves, which in some cases is good, and in a lot of cases is not very helpful. This is because any belief about ourselves is a limit that ultimately must be broken.

All too often we pigeon-hole ourselves, saying things like, "I've always been this way," "Oh, that always makes me so mad," "That's just the way I've always felt," and so on.

But in fact the only thing we've always been and always will be is infinite creative energy, free to be whatever we choose.

To understand how to change an old fear program it is helpful to think of the brain as a computer. What you feed into it determines what it gives out. If you program in worry, confusion, and fear it will manifest experiences for you that conform to your programming. But if you change the program, expecting the best, affirming your creative ability, worthiness and success, the old programs will lose all their energy and no longer affect your life.

We have given ourselves so many debilitating programs that we shouldn't wonder why we have so many physical and mental ills. We are constantly saying things like I'm confused, I'm stupid, I'm too fat, I'm sick and tired of so and so, I'll never forgive myself, I just hate that s.o.b., and so on. And these are just the little minor ones that plague our systems every day.

A pattern of hatred, grief, rejection, irritability, or whatever held in the mind long enough becomes the dominant thought pattern. Finally we believe that it is the only reality. We are so locked into our own negative creations, entrenched in a rut, that we don't escape. In fact we learn to like our rut, because it's comfortable, something familiar. We get a false sense of security from it.

But year after year can you imagine what holding hurts, griefs and negativity does to your system? (Some estimate that over 70 percent of our thoughts are negative!) Not only does this eat away at your body, slowly destroying healthful functioning, but it also destroys your brain cells and ability to think clearly.

Holding on to negative thoughts is one of the reasons we grow old and senile. There is no reason we should not become stronger with age. The body could easily last from 150 to 200 years without the stress and negativity we subject it to. As we continue to advance in medical science and build immunities to virtually all known diseases, the last and chief offender will be our own life style, the way we think and feel about ourselves and others.

Aging, a Negative Program

Many people I counsel with are afraid of growing older. Many of us have been programmed by our culture that youth is beauty, strength and health, and that when one's youth begins to fade he slowly becomes debilitated.

A certain sadness begins to set in with many people with the passing of physical youth. We begin to look at gray hair, wrinkles, and let the build up of concerns and worries take their toll on our energy.

It is extremely important that we guard against identifying with the programming, "I am growing old." If we dwell on outer appearances, we lose an inner awareness of vitality and strength. Part of our life task here on the earth plane is to learn to look within instead of without. Age should impart strength, not frailty; wisdom, not senility.

There is no such thing as age in the realms of spirit. When we begin to nurture the spirit of life within ourselves we truly find the Power that does not know age, sickness or frustration. We find that this power, when awakened, can revitalize us moment by moment.

You are spirit—you don't *have* a spirit, you *are* a spirit, an energy being. When we are around those rare souls who have learned to identify with the true self, we sense a special kind of presence. For these persons seem to radiate a timelessness, an eternal quality of beauty. Their inner being, not outer appearances, has become their reality. They see through the images of time, and are grounded in what has been called the eternal now.

An ancient Chinese proverb says, "A long life is only the blink of an eye." We put so much emphasis on *years*, rather than on qualities of awareness.

If we would discover inner peace and harmony, if we would truly know the eternal quality of youth, we must change our perspective on who we are. We must refocus our awareness on the inner reality.

If we seek to identify with the material world, the mirror of life will reflect our own mortality and temporal nature. If we identify with the inner spiritual reality, the mirror will reflect an eternal process of growth.

The spirit of youth is the spirit of creativity. Perhaps you have heard the saying that we grow old when we cease to dream new dreams. To continuously awaken to new joy, new vitality and wisdom is the name of the game if we would experience that elusive quality called youth.

To help rejuvenate your awareness, and consequently rejuvenate your body, mind and spirit, each day remember these four words: *In the beginning God. . . .* The creative spirit is the ever beginning, never ending life force. Each day our lives should mark a new beginning in understanding and harmony. Day by day we can open ourselves to new awareness, which will empower and invigorate us. It is only our negative thinking and identification with the time-space world that robs us of our natural spiritual growth into greater strength as the physical years go by.

Emotional Trauma and Mental Illness

Emotional problems, whether mild or major, are the result of low energy and running negative programs. What we call mental illness, which is a more developed stage of emotional unrest, results from not understanding how to use and direct energy. People are labeled and put into many different categories—psychotic, neurotic, schizophrenic, manic-depressive, and so on—but very little is understood about treating the mentally ill.

Except in cases where there is severe brain damage, virtually all mental illness can be overcome. It is difficult to do, however, when a patient is kept on tranquilizers or severely drugged.

A person playing the mentally ill role has on some level made the decision to do this. Perhaps it is a fear of responsibility, a vie for attention, or ignorance of the energy system. I have worked with so-called mental patients, and find one of several things to be true.

Playing the Game

First, there are those who are playing the game. They have all the symptoms and may be committed to an institution.

I was asked by a doctor to interview a young boy who was in a mental institution to determine whether he could be helped. I went in and talked with him about 20 minutes, read him up one side and down the other, and then asked why he was playing the role. He said that everything I had told him was correct, but that if he got well he would have to accept too much responsibility. He didn't want to do that. It was easier to be mentally ill, to be taken care of. (People level with me because they know I can tune in to where they are really at.)

So I had to tell the doctors that they might as well forget it for awhile, because this young man did not choose to get well. I told the patient, however, to come and see me when he decided to get out, because I felt it would just be a matter of time until he tired of what he was doing.

Another time a woman came in for a reading bringing her psychologist and live-in aid with her. She was supposed to be so sick that she couldn't live alone. She began to tell me about all her mental problems, her neuroses, and manic-depressive personality. She threw herself on the floor and cried for a few minutes. She seemed to delight in putting on quite a show.

I asked her how long she was going to continue this farce, and she sat up in shocked recognition of her game. But within the next few minutes she was back into it again. She didn't want to give it up because she thought she had too much to lose. Her psychologist smiled knowingly, also realizing she was playing a game.

It turned out that she was doing this to punish her wealthy parents, who could afford to give her all the psychologists and treatment she wanted. She thought they had never loved her, and this was her way of forcing them to be concerned and give her attention.

We have a lot invested in our neuroses and psychoses. We have discovered they give us certain rewards that we think are satisfying. Although mental institutions don't realize it, they most often perpetuate the behavior they supposedly want to remedy, because they reinforce it. There are those in the medical profession who believe that mental illness is a self-inflicted myth, and this comes very close to the truth.

Too Wide Open

Next, there is the problem of those souls who are very sensitive to energy and don't know how to control it. They are so wide open that their energy goes up and down—the typical manic-depressive syndrome—depending upon who they are around and what their thoughts happen to be at the moment. They don't know how to tune out other people.

I retreated from the world for five years when I was a teenager because I didn't know how to tune other people out. I would be walking down the street, picking up everyone else's trips, getting depressed, not knowing where it was coming from. I couldn't go to movies because I would get paranoid and have to leave. As I would begin concentrating on the screen I would open myself up, and would pick up all the negativity of those around me.

So one has to learn how to say, "Hey, wait a minute. Is this my trip or somebody else's?" One has to learn how to build up the energy field in order to cope. We've got enough of our own trips without having to be concerned with those everybody else is running.

Through meditation and positive programming you can build up the energy field and learn not to react to every thought you pick up. (Sensitive people can also help stabilize their energy by eating every two and a half hours.)

All the counseling in the world won't help correct a problem unless the person is working on building his energy. This is why there is no evidence that psychotherapy works any faster or better than not having any therapy at all. You can spend months looking for reasons for your condition, analyzing your background, blaming circumstances in your life, but until you get your energy up your perception and condition won't change.

The Psychics

There are also people who are extremely psychic and don't understand how to shut off this heightened sensitivity. They really hear voices and see other beings, but when they tell the doctor about it he says they are hallucinating. The schizophrenic, for example, doesn't know how to tune out. The psychic level of awareness is very real, separated from ordinary reality by but a thin veil.

This is what the psychic tunes in to, picking up information about people, seeing their guides and teachers. But no one can stay tuned in all the time or he will have a nervous breakdown, lose his sense of control and self-awareness.

When I go to lectures or give readings I tune into my channel, which actually extends beyond the psychic into the intuitive level of awareness. I hear things, feel things, sometimes I see things, and I am given information about others to help them with their problems. This is coming from my higher intuition, a higher level of reality. When I leave my office or the lecture hall, I tune out. I change from the intuitive channel back into the person Betty. I can listen when I want to listen, and shut it off when I don't want to.

This again is the importance of learning to close down. When you have a heightened energy field you begin picking up more and more frequencies. This is to your advantage as long as you know that you are in control. But we must learn to tune in to one thing or person at a time. Otherwise it is like listening to hundreds of different radio channels at once, so the messages are garbled and often frightening.

People need to understand that there are many realities, and you might get messages from many different levels of your being. But you are in control, and nothing can go against your free will unless you deliberately give it up. You can tell any voice, image, entity or thought form to go away, to go to progression, and it must leave. This means that the entity must continue on to a higher level, progress to another dimension where it can learn instead of play tricks on or pester people.

Possession

Another level of mental disturbance results from actually being possessed by another entity. This happens when a person gives up control of his body through extremely low or scattered energy. It happens to alcoholics when they have a personality change after a few drinks. They have lost control, and another entity has just moved in.

These aren't evil entities, just lower level ignorant beings who don't know any better. Shock treatments can serve the purpose of ejecting an entity so that the person who really lives in the body can come back. Unfortunately the effects of shock treatments don't last because the person does nothing to keep his energy up, and unfortunately they burn out your brain cells.

You yourself can eject an entity by standing behind the patient, placing the thumbs on either side of the spinal column or the back of the neck with the fingers resting beside the collar bone. Take a deep breath, and as you exhale imagine energy flowing through you into the person, moving up and down the spine. (This technique is the basic laying on of hands given in Chapter 5.) The energy jolt will have the same results as the shock treatment, but with no bad side effects.

You should also realize that automatic writing and Ouija boards are not games, but open you up to possible exploitation by other entities. When you allow another entity to use your hand you are beginning to give up control. I never recommend that you work with Ouija boards or automatic writing because it can lead to many dangerous experiences. I have seen many women in mental hospitals who have wound up there as a direct result of automatic writing. *NEVER* give over control of your physical body to anyone. Don't be gullible. Be an open-minded skeptic and you'll stay balanced and in total control at all times. You can get any answers you want through meditation, and always maintain your control.

The automatic writing and Ouija board business is part of the astral plane or psychic phenomena level, and it is kindergarten stuff. It is not something to fool around with. You want to go beyond the psychic and use your higher intuition, and this is done through expanding your own consciousness, not listening to whatever wants to come through you. Any teacher or entity that tells you how to live your life is not a high teacher. You can get general insight, but must learn to make your own mistakes and follow your own intuition. Otherwise, you aren't growing.

The earth plane is our school. It provides us with tests which are opportunities to grow and learn. If we always had the answers given to us, what would we learn? Life is simple! We just need the eyes to see and the ears to hear.

Disease, an Imbalance

Whether we experience disease as physical or mental illness, as minor or major, it is always brought on by our attitudes and ways of living. There is no such thing as a "big killer disease" that is out to get us. We develop great fear of some diseases, such as heart trouble and cancer, but these are no more difficult to correct than any other if we understand that we have created them and we can change them.

It is not infrequent that a person is told that he has a terminal disease and just so many months to live. Often, if these persons suddenly decide to do everything they always wanted to do, to get as much in as possible in the remaining time, the terminal illness vanishes. For once they are responding to their inner feelings and leadings, functioning in harmony with themselves.

We can learn to take control of our physical systems and our mental-emotional systems, restoring perfect balance and harmony. The first step is accepting responsibility for our lives, and then learning to keep our energy high and let go of fears and negative programming. Nothing ever changes except our perception—we are forever tuning into levels of harmony or disharmony, balance or imbalance, health or disease.

Decide to choose health, sanity and balance, and you will find your life becomes transformed!

Chapter 4

Healing Yourself

You Deserve Health

Self-healing really involves learning to love yourself. It means loving the God-self within, and recognizing that the natural state of your being is health and harmony. It is your right to be healthy, harmonious and happy in every area of your life. You deserve it. But you must realize you deserve it, and be willing to let go of any and all of the old programs and habit patterns of negativity that stand in your way.

You might say, "But God knows I want to be healthy. Why doesn't He just make me well and bring me happiness?" God may know all of your needs, but *you* have to know in order to manifest them. That is what prayer is all about. It's up to you to identify the problem and know what you need to correct it in order to manifest it in your experience. You have to ask to receive. In other words, God offers the gift of perfect health, but you must ask for it, accept it, and claim it as your own.

The Most Effective Tools

There are many techniques you can use to begin a total balancing and harmonizing of your system. The most effective tools are relaxation, meditation, affirmation and visualization. Relaxation is listed here first, because without learning to relax, you cannot meditate, you are not open to receiving positive affirmations, and your efforts at visualization will be difficult. You must be relaxed both to send and receive the healing energy.

With each of these tools you are opening to your natural reservoir of healing energy, creating new thought patterns that allow this energy to flow smoothly and harmoniously throughout your physical, mental and spiritual being. You have all the energy and inner wisdom you need to bring about a perfect healing within you, but often the problem lies in convincing yourself of this fact. For so long we have not accepted responsibility for our health!

Relaxation

Most illnesses would be eliminated if people knew how to relax. When you are deeply relaxed all levels of your being are resonating in harmony. Relaxation helps you return to the basic simplicity of your being, a level of insight in which you are calm and centered. It helps you focus on the infinite energy reservoir within you, rather than focusing on the struggle and confusion that so often seems to thrive around you.

Relaxation is an attitude of being, a state of mind and body which is in harmony with the world around you. Learning to deeply relax physically is the first step toward creating this inner awareness of well-being, because as you consciously let go of physical tension, mental and emotional tension also fall away. It is impossible to be deeply physically relaxed and remain mentally uptight!

Meditation

Meditation helps you center your energies, heighten your awareness and expand your energy field. It recharges your batteries by channeling energy through your system, cleanses the chakras, awakens the kundalini, and helps you maintain an objective detachment so you can look at the numbers you're running.

Daily meditation is your best insurance against poor health, because you can look at emotional reactions as they arise, ask for insight on problems day by day, and clear out a great deal of mental clutter in a very short time. A person who is meditating can move through the equivalence of several lifetimes in one, because our awareness and self-growth greatly increases. Deep meditation also includes deep relaxation, harmonizing and aligning the energies of your system.

Affirmation

The words that you think and speak have great power. To affirm something means to make firm, to strengthen. Whatever you affirm through your words becomes true in your life. The negative power of words constantly manifests in our affairs, and through criticism, unforgiveness, and self-depreciation we continuously bring various diseases upon ourselves.

When we begin to use the positive power of affirmations, affirming health and wholeness, vitality and prosperity, we can change the whole pattern and direction of our life and health. Perhaps you have tried using affirmations, thinking, "Oh yes, that's just positive thinking," and it didn't really work. But to be effective affirmations must be used every day, again and again, until they have totally dislodged the negative. We must withdraw all of the energy we have invested in our negativity and critical attitudes, and reinvest it in loving, supportive, life-affirming attitudes.

Visualization

You have often heard that a picture is worth a thousand words. If we can communicate thought pictures of health and harmony to our system, it will conform to the image. Through the use of visual imagery, or your imagination, you can deliberately direct energy throughout your body and focus on specific areas or concerns to hasten the healing process.

When you imagine your body filling with energy, this is in fact happening. When you imagine a white light engulfing you, it is really there. Your imagination is the door to God consciousness, because it puts you in touch with your infinite creative ability to direct energy and manifest whatever you want in your life. But it is important to get control of our thought pictures, because a negative image of the self held in the mind will manifest just as quickly as a positive one. If the inner picture we hold of ourselves is one of helplessness and despondency, then our outer actions will conform to this. We can create our self-image, our good health and harmonious relations with others when we realize that we have this power and, in fact, are already using it unknowingly for better or for worse.

The techniques given in this chapter combine all of the above. Remember that they are devices for getting in touch with and effectively directing your own life force or healing energy. You may improvise and develop techniques of your own. You may wish to record one or two that you use the most on a cassette, so that you can relax totally and follow it along. Be sure to use a positive and loving voice.

A suggested schedule might be the following: meditate once a day, either morning or evening, and before you close down at the end of meditation practice the visualizations or repeat the affirmations you are working with. Before going to sleep at night, do an overall body relaxation, releasing the tensions of the day. Never go to sleep feeling anxious or worried, but instead forgive yourself and others for anything that may have happened during the day, and close your eyes feeling at peace with the world.

For meditation practice to really begin to stabilize your energy about two or three years are needed. To move beyond physical sickness, to be free from disease, about 20 years are necessary. But you will begin to feel almost immediate results in calming and centering your thoughts. When using positive affirmations and visualization, you should allow from three to six weeks before evaluating the results, because time is needed for the new programs to take a firm hold in your thought patterns.

Don't try to use will power when doing the techniques, but relax in an effortless way and let the visualizations and affirmations flow gently into your mind. Expect them to work for you, and don't worry every two or three days about whether anything is happening. These are powerful tools, and they have powerful effects! Some healings are instantaneous, and others take more time. So relax and flow with what is happening.

Relaxation Techniques

Tense-Relax. This technique is designed to loosen the tension in your muscles and totally relax the body. It should be done lying down, without any restrictive or tight clothing on, and is excellent right before going to sleep at night.

1. Inhale and exhale deeply several times, consciously letting go of all the tension in your body. Close your eyes.

2. Beginning with your toes, you are going to direct your attention to the different areas of your body, tensing them, releasing the tension, and relaxing completely. Tense the toes and feet, point the toes up or down, feel the increase in tension, take a deep breath, then exhale and let the tension go.

3. Direct your attention to your lower legs, knees, and thighs. Tense these muscles, feel the tension, take a deep breath, then exhale and let the tension go completely.

4. Continue in the same way by directing your attention to the buttocks, lower back, upper back and shoulders, each time tensing the muscles, feeling the tension, inhaling, then exhaling completely and releasing the tension.

5. Direct your attention to the hands and fingers, lower arms, elbows and upper arms. Tighten the muscles by making a fist with your hands, stiffening the arms and raising them to about a 45 degree angle. Feel the tension, take a deep breath, exhale and release the tension completely.

6. Continue in the same way to direct your attention to your abdomen, stomach and chest muscles. Tense each muscle group, feel the tension, inhale deeply and then exhale and release the tension.

7. Be aware of the muscles in your neck, head and face. Tense these muscles, stiffening the neck and making a big grimace on the face. Feel the tension, inhale, then exhale and release the tension.

8. Now tighten every muscle in your body, imagining that you are becoming stiff and rigid like a board. Feel the tension all over, inhale and increase the tension, exhale and release the tension completely.

9. Relax, breathing normally, mentally repeating the following: "I am relaxing my entire body. All tension is melting away. My body and mind are completely renewed and rejuvenated."

10. If you are going to sleep, give yourself the suggestion that when you awaken you will be refreshed and filled with vitality. If you are going to get up and continue with your daily activities, suggest to yourself that when you open your eyes you will feel rested and fully awake, eager to continue with your tasks.

(Every night before I go to sleep I do the tense-relax, and this releases any tension that I may have built up during the day. When I started this a few years ago I suddenly discovered that I slept much better, and no longer woke up with a crick in my neck or with sore muscles from tension that had been hanging on from the day before. I highly recommend it.)

Quick Tense-Relax. Whenever you feel tension in any area of your body you can direct your awareness to the area, deliberately increase the tension by tightening the muscles, and then let it go. This works especially well with tension built up in the neck and shoulders. Also, for an instant all over relaxer, tighten all the muscles in your body, becoming stiff and rigid (step 8 in the above), inhale, feel the tension, then exhale and let the tension go.

Neck Rolls. Neck rolls also can aid in the reduction of tension and eyestrain, and can be done while sitting at your desk or riding on a bus. Imagine your neck is limp, then gently and slowly roll your head around to the right shoulder, back, left shoulder and front. Repeat several times in each direction.

Focusing on the Breath. Breath is an important regulator of energy in the body. Whenever you feel nervous or uptight, focus on your breathing, just watching the breath flow in and out of your body. As you inhale mentally repeat, "I am . . ." and as you exhale mentally repeat, ". . . relaxed." By attuning to "I am . . . relaxed" for a few moments you will experience immediate calming effects.

The Inner Light Foundation Meditation Technique

This meditation technique was given to me by my channel, and is an ancient Egyptian method. It is very simple yet very effective, and is divided into two parts: concentration and meditation. (Remember that any meditation technique is good as long as you remember to close down at the end of it.)

During meditation you are expanding your energy field, heightening your senses, and at the end you should close down. Closing down doesn't mean you are shutting off awareness of other people or your awareness of the inner self. It involves putting a protective sphere of energy around you so that you can maintain high energy without getting it drained off, prevent negativity from coming into your field, and stabilize your own system.

To do this you simply imagine that you are surrounded in a huge circle or balloon of light. This is the white light energy of love. You then close the palms of your hands and open your eyes.

You can imagine yourself in this protective white light at any time during the day, whether or not you have just meditated, and it will serve to heighten your energy and center your thoughts. The white light is a real and dynamic force, and when you imagine it around you it is really there. Thoughts are things!

Also, if your energy suddenly drops you can just take three deep breaths, turn your palms up to receive energy and mentally holler, "Help!" You'll feel a new surge of energy filling you, for your teachers walking with you will always come to your aid. Then picture the white light around you and close your palms.

Protecting your energy is just as important as building it, so don't forget to use the white light as a valuable tool.

The meditation technique is given again here as it is in all of my books, because it is the foundation of all the teachings. There are seven basic steps:

1. Sit in a straight back chair with spine erect, feet flat on the floor. Fold your hands together in your lap, or hold them in prayer position. Your eyes may be opened or closed. (If you prefer to sit in a lotus position with legs crossed, fine.)

2. Take several deep breaths, and feel yourself relaxing. Imagine a bright white light completely surrounding you, which is your protection as you open sensitive energy centers.

3. Gently concentrate on a single idea, picture or word for about ten minutes. Select something that suggests peace, beauty, or a spiritual ideal. (Keep the same object of concentration throughout a given concentration period.) You may choose to play soft, soothing music during this time, and focus your concentration by listening to it.

4. If your mind strays from your object of concentration, gently bring it back to your focal point. (Don't criticize yourself for wandering, just become aware of it and return as often as you need to the concentration object. Surprisingly soon you'll find your ability to discipline the mind growing much stronger.)

5. After about 10 minutes separate your hands and turn them palms up in your lap. Close your eyes if opened.

6. Relax your hold on the concentration object, and shift your mind into neutral. Remain passive yet alert for 10 minutes. Placidly observe any thoughts and images as they come and go. Just be still, detached, and flow with whatever you are experiencing.

7. After about 10 minutes open your eyes, close your palms, and again imagine that you are surrounded completely by a white light. This is your continued protection as you go about your daily activities.

This twenty minute period is all that is necessary to recharge your energy field each day. But we should continue to practice the meditative attitude throughout the day, watching our thoughts and behavior, observing in a detached way how we are setting up our own experiences. Remember meditation is not an escape from life, but an orientation which allows us to be more fully involved in our own growth process. And it will definitely change your life, because it changes you.

If you want to send healing energy to yourself or others or include visualization or positive affirmations in your meditation period, it is most effective to practice them at the close of step 6, before closing down and opening your eyes.

Affirmations for Health

As suggested before, affirmations are easy to use when you record them on a cassette tape so you can play them whenever you want, relaxing completely and listening to their meaning. But you can also read them to yourself, or memorize them and repeat them whenever you wish.

You are most receptive to positive affirmations when you are deeply relaxed, and it is especially helpful to use them before going to sleep at night and when you first wake up in the morning. You should repeat each one at least twice, getting into the feeling of the affirmation as much as possible. The following are suggested for health and well-being, and you should put them in your own words so they feel comfortable when you say them:

1. The natural state of my being is health, harmony and wholeness.

2. My mind is in every cell of my body, and it builds and adjusts according to my thinking and feeling.

3. My body is energy, fluid and pliable, and my positive thoughts move easily through it to create perfect health.

4. I am in control of my life and my health. I choose health, harmony and wholeness.

5. My body, mind and spirit are in complete harmony at all times. I maintain balance in physical, mental, emotional and spiritual states of my being.

6. I am filled with energy, vitality, and radiant health.

7. I am now recognizing and correcting all limiting beliefs that stand in the way of my health and happiness.

8. There is nothing to fear. I am free to create whatever I desire.

9. My mind is adjusting my body metabolism to achieve and maintain my ideal weight.

10. Universal love flows through my body, mind and spirit. Every cell and tissue, thought and memory, is balanced and harmonized in love.

11. I greet all persons with unconditional love. Love dissolves all hate, fear, anxiety and insecurity which cause imbalance in my life.

12. I see myself as a unique individual with a special purpose to fulfill in this lifetime. I am gaining clear insight on what my purpose is and I am being directed toward my life goal.

13. I am learning to love and respect myself more and more each day.

14. My life cannot be limited. I am free to manifest my infinite potential now.

15. I recognize that pain is a signal of disharmony. If pain manifests I immediately correct all disharmony within my physical, mental and emotional organism.

You should choose perhaps five or six affirmations to work with at a time. And, you can reprogram any fear or anxiety simply by focusing on the positive instead of the negative. For example, if you think you're too selfish, affirm: "I am developing an increasing love for others." If you have a fear of speaking before groups, affirm: "I am developing more and more confidence in my speaking ability, looking forward to opportunities to interact with new people." If you are afraid of failure, repeat: "My success is assured." Always replace a negative with a positive.

Visualization Techniques

A Healthy Self-Image. It is important to have a basic image in your mind of yourself as a happy and healthy individual. If you have low energy at present, or are suffering from some particular ailment, picture yourself in vigorous health doing something that suggests vitality and well-being. You may be climbing a mountain, hiking, playing tennis, jogging on the beach, or whatever you choose. At the close of each meditation period, or before going to sleep at night, bring this picture of radiant health to your mental screen, and feel and sense it with your whole being. Smell the fragrance in the air, feel the clothes you are wearing, and become one with the image as best you can. Then release it from your mind, mentally repeating or saying aloud, "I deserve it and it is so."

You can also use the positive image technique for changing unwanted habits. For example, if you want to stop smoking, dwell on an image of yourself as a non-smoker. See yourself feeling wonderful, talking with friends, perfectly relaxed and confident, minus the cigarettes. Picture yourself saying, "I no longer have any desire for cigarettes, and am enjoying being a non-smoker." Imagine one of your friends congratulating you on kicking the habit. Every time you light up a cigarette, flash this image of yourself as a non-smoker on your mental screen, and it will gradually begin to take over as your new reality.

You can use this technique with weight loss—picturing yourself as your ideal weight, with a drinking problem, insomnia, or whatever. Remember: never dwell on an image of yourself as sick, fearful, or confused. Our present behavior is the result of the self-images we hold, whether conscious or subconscious, and we are free to change any of them we do not want. The key to success is continuous use of the positive images, especially when we find ourselves engaged in the habit we wish to break.

Loving Your Body. Many people do not like their physical vehicles. Perhaps they think they are too fat, too skinny, too short, too tall, too busty, not busty enough, or out of proportion in one way or another. When we reject any part of ourselves, and think we are physically ugly, we are not sending love to our bodies. Over a period of time this negative thinking toward your body results in disease.

We have been programmed with many images of what the body beautiful should look like. But no two bodies are the same, nor should they be. Remember: you chose the body you inhabit, and it is up to you to love it and take care of it. And the amazing thing is, the more you learn to love your body for just what it is, the more beautiful it becomes.

It is the inner beauty that transforms the outer appearance. People don't love you because of your body, but because of what radiates from within. They are attracted by your vibrations, not your physical appearance.

Take some time to become aware of your body, to appreciate it, for the magnificent vehicle that it is. Get in a comfortable and relaxed position, and then beginning with your toes, consciously direct your attention to every area of your body, talking to and loving each part. Then closing your eyes, imagine that you are taking a journey through the inside of your body, visiting all the organs, muscles, bones, the nervous system, circulatory system, and so on. Talk to your cells and tissues, acknowledging their intelligence and energy, and imagine you are sending love to them, honoring them for the part they play in your total body-mind-spirit being.

You will be amazed at the wonderful rejuvenating effect this will have on you, and you will begin to appreciate yourself more as a total energy system.

Self-Healing through Color. Color is a dynamic force in healing. Different colors have different healing properties. One can use a specific color for specific ailments, but you can always use the white light energy which contains all the colors of the spectrum.

All colors are valuable to our well-being, and often we choose a particular color to wear on a certain day. If we are low energy, for example, we might choose red. If we feel nervous or hyperactive, we might choose blue or purple. Parents should also be sensitive to the colors their children choose, and not try to dress them in something they don't feel comfortable with. Probably their system is rejecting the color because it needs something else.

A helpful visualization technique involves imagining all the colors of the rainbow moving up the spine, balancing and harmonizing all the energy centers of the body. It is good for cleansing and balancing.

1. Sit in the meditation position, breath deeply and begin to relax. Consciously relax all the tension within your body.

2. Be aware of the position of your body, then become aware of your extended energy field. Remind yourself that your body is energy, and that you are now going to harmonize all energy centers through directing the healing properties of color throughout your system.

3. Direct your attention to the base of your spine, the root chakra. Imagine a disc of pulsating, vibrating red light energy forming at the base of your spine. Expand the disc, extending it into a band of color interpenetrating your body from front to back, extending into your energy field. Feel the special healing properties of the red. Then gradually float the band of color up the spine about two inches.

4. Now return your attention to the base of the spine again, and picture a disc of orange light. Imagine this disc spreading out, interpenetrating your being from front to back, extending into your energy field, aligning itself beneath the red band of color. Imagine both colors moving together up the spine another two inches.

5. Return your attention to the base of the spine again, and picture a yellow disc of light. Continue with the same process, in turn picturing green, blue, indigo and violet. Then you have a rainbow of colors effortlessly moving up the spine, and each energy center is taking exactly what it needs from each color to restore perfect functioning.

6. Float the rainbow out the top of your head, and let all the colors blend into a bright sun of white light

energy about six inches above the head. Then expand the sun of white light until it engulfs your entire being, becoming the protective white light encircling you.

Cleansing the System. Visualization conveys a message to the deeper levels of your being: to restore, correct imbalances, eliminate disease of all kinds. One highly popular and effective technique is designed to work with particular areas of your body that need healing.

1. Sit in the meditation position, breath deeply and relax.
2. If there is a particular area of your body that is diseased, picture this area in a certain way: as grey, red, etc., as being inhabited by miniature villains (complete with masks and guns) or whatever you wish to create in your imagination. This helps you identify a problem area, get hold of it, recognize and work with it. You become more fully involved in the exercise.
3. Now recreate the sun of energy over your head. Expand the sun until it is two or three feet in diameter, and feel its intensity.
4. Imagine the sun is opening up, and an unlimited supply of its liquid light energy begins to flood through your being. Picture and feel this stream of energy flowing into your head, neck and shoulders, down through your chest and abdomen, down your back and out the soles of your feet, down your arms and out the palms of your hands, flooding into your energy field.
5. See this energy completely washing away the color you pictured (chasing the villains away, etc.). Imagine your entire being as radiant energy, all disharmony washed completely out of your body and energy field.
6. Now again return your awareness to the sun of energy over your head. Again expand it to completely

surround and engulf you, becoming the protective white light. Mentally affirm: "My body, mind and spirit are renewed in health and wholeness."

(This technique is also effective for getting rid of headaches. Locate the headache, picture it as a color, then wash it out of your system.)

Emotional Healing. As I have already emphasized, we will never be rid of disharmony until we remove the *cause* behind it. Two of the most important emotional healers, responsible for the elimination of much of what we call disease, are forgiveness and release. When you forgive yourself or others, you are reestablishing peace and harmony within, eliminating negativity, guilt and hostility.

To *for give* is to give something for. You are giving yourself love instead of condemnation, giving others understanding rather than hostility and anger. Remember that every experience you have ever had is for your learning and is positive, and that no one can hurt you unless you choose to be hurt. We must look at all experiences and ask ourselves: What is the lesson for me here? Then thank the person or persons involved for helping you to learn more about yourself.

We are all going to make mistakes, no one here on the earth plane is perfect. We must realize that each being is a fellow God-child, who in his own way is growing toward realizing the God within. The best way for us to help others grow, and to help ourselves grow, is to learn from and move beyond what we call negative experiences. It only slows us down to carry around grudges, guilts and disappointments.

One of the problems in not being able to forgive others is that we think they have taken something away from us: self-esteem, love, money, a job, a lover, and so on. Perhaps we think they tricked us, took advantage of us. Again, we would be angry because we think we lost our sense of self-worth.

The fact is that no one can take anything away from you unless you give it to them. And no one can give you anything if you don't accept it.

The following technique combines visualization and affirmation, and can be used with any person or situation that you need to forgive:

1. Relax your body and mind, breathe deeply, and close your eyes.

2. Imagine that you are in a beautiful setting, at the mountains, the beach, walking along a forest trail. You feel completely relaxed and at peace with yourself.

3. Now picture the person you have not forgiven walking toward you. You see this person as a fellow radiant being, walking through life working on lessons just like you are. You walk up, face the person and affirm: "I completely and fully forgive you, and you completely and fully forgive me. All disharmony between us melts away. I let go of all resentment and grudges, and you let go of all resentment and grudges. We are each free to follow our highest good now."

4. If you feel this person took something away from you (for example, your self-esteem), imagine him handing you a package that says "My Self-Esteem" on it. Picture him saying, "Here you are. I never wanted this package, but you gave it to me. I'm glad to give it back." Then imagine the package turning into energy, and merging with your being.

5. Then imagine each of you surrounded in the white light of love, smiling at one another, and then turn and walk away.

(It may take several weeks before you begin to feel like you want to forgive a particular person or situation. But you will finally break through the resistance, and the negative energy you have bottled up inside will melt away. And when one person forgives, this starts an automatic response with the other person involved. Forgiveness becomes a mutual and supportive interaction.)

The following affirmation is especially helpful to use every night right before going to sleep. Simply affirm in a state of deep relaxation: "I forgive everyone, everything, every experience, every memory and every thought that needs forgiveness. I freely and completely forgive, and I am freely and completely forgiven. Universal Love is now adjusting and harmonizing my life, and I am filled with peace."

Then feel a deep sense of peace enveloping you, and enter your sleep state in harmony with the world.

Forgiveness is a perfect way to relax mentally, physically and spiritually, letting the love force flow through your being to heal all disharmony. Love is not a corrector, but a transformer. It is not the way of an eye for an eye and a tooth for a tooth. It is a totally new way of seeing yourself and your fellows, and responding from this higher perspective that all of us are cosmic beings, temporarily residing on this planet to learn a thing or two.

Besides being willing to forgive ourselves and others, we must also learn to release our tense hold on people and events. We cling to others, especially our children and loved ones, wanting them to conform to our expectations, afraid we will lose them. We forget that each one of us must find his own way, and that the Cosmic Intelligence, God's will, flows through all lives.

What is truly yours is impossible to lose. What truly belongs to you will always return. We must learn to relax, release, and flow with life, trusting ourselves and the God-force within all beings.

We must also release our hold on experiences, events, and many of our ideas of security. The only security or permanence we will ever know is the inner security of who we are—infinite creative energy. Everything else changes, nothing is ever the same. If we focus on the phenomena in the outer world, we will never see truth behind the fluctuation and temporariness. If we focus on the inner self, we will begin to see the thread of reality weaving all experiences on the same loom.

Releasing others is a wonderful emotional stabilizer. The following exercise works in the same way as the five step forgiveness technique above, changing the affirmation in Step 3 as follows: "I freely and completely release you, and you freely and completely release me. We are each free to follow our highest leading, and Universal Love directs each life to its perfect fulfillment now."

Another powerful release affirmation is the following: "I let go of my possessive attitudes toward people, events, ideas and things. That which I willingly release to God I never lose, for that or something better always flows into my life in return. Releasing enables me to flow with the natural, harmonious Life Energy, producing perfect results in health, happiness and fulfillment."

Calming the Emotions. Whenever you feel uptight a quick calming technique is often the key to get you through a particular situation. Close your eyes and visualize an inner pool or lake, and observe what it looks like. If the water is choppy or wavy, imagine that you are spreading your hand across the lake and stilling the waters, calming the turmoil. Your emotional state will calm down in the process. Or if the lake you visualize is clear and peaceful, simply dwell on that image and allow the serenity to spread throughout your body and mind.

If you suddenly feel beset by problems coming at you from all directions, imagine yourself as a giant rock, with sea waves crashing all around you. The waves may break over you, but you are firm and strong and can ride out any storm. Then imagine that the sea around you is quieting down, and you see clearly in all directions. Your perception is enhanced, and you know exactly what steps to take to handle any and all situations.

Visualizing Your Teacher. This exercise can be used to receive insight on many different problems, such as the cause of a disease, new healthful attitudes you might adopt, insight into relationships, and so on. The basic idea is to relax and imagine that you are meeting a wise teacher, enlightened being, or your own higher self. You talk with this being, ask questions, and in answer the being may give you a gift (which is symbolic of your answer), verbally explain the situation to you, or help you understand what you seek in another meaningful way. It is a process to tap into your own inner wisdom, which already knows the answer to all problems, the cure for every ailment, and the best direction for your life. The steps are as follows:

1. Relax in a meditative position and close your eyes.

2. Imagine that you are walking down a path, lush vegetation all around you. The farther you go, the more relaxed you feel. This path is taking you to a very beautiful and special place (wherever you choose: atop a mountain, beside a lake, to a meadow).

3. You arrive at your special place, feeling at one with yourself and at peace with the world around you. You find a comfortable spot and settle down. In the distance you notice a light moving toward you, and you become aware immediately of a strong feeling of love, realizing that this is the light of a wonderful teacher.

4. The teacher approaches and you greet one another in love and joy, relaxing together for a few moments. Then you ask the teacher a particular question

you have, the more specific the better, and wait for the reply. It may be in the form of a symbol, gesture, words or an inner knowing.

5. You thank your teacher for joining you, bid farewell, and turn to walk back down the path taking the new insight with you.

Another form of this visualization of higher teachers is the following: Relax and close your eyes, then imagine a semi-circle of teachers dressed in white standing before you. Imagine all of them with their arms outstretched in love toward your third eye, pouring energy into your being. Relax and experience this energy flooding into your body, mind and spirit for a few minutes.

This exercise provides an immediate boost of love energy and support, and develops the inner knowing that you are never alone, but surrounded by an unseen brotherhood of higher beings.

Self-Healing Through Dreams

Dreams are a special level of inner visualization and insight and are a valuable tool in problem solving. You can learn to program your dreams to give you the answer to any concern you might have. Great discoveries have come through the dream state throughout the ages, and this source of inner guidance and help is available to each one of us.

Dreams give us a reading on where we are physically, mentally and spiritually. In order to gain control and understanding of dreams you should first begin remembering and writing them down, and then move on to problem solving. Everyone dreams, whether you remember dreaming or not, and with the following technique you can begin to recall them:

To practice remembering a dream, sit on the side of your bed right before going to sleep, breath deeply and relax. Then say to yourself: "Tonight I want to remember a dream, and I *will* remember a dream. As soon as I awaken I will write it down." Then go to sleep with a pad and pencil beside your bed, expecting to remember and write down a dream as soon as you awaken. (If you prefer, record your dream into a cassette recorder.)

After you are reliably remembering your dreams for three and four nights in a row, use the dream state for problem solving by programming the following right before going to bed: "Tonight I will have and remember a dream containing information for the solution of this problem. The problem concerns . . . (and briefly describe it as objectively as possible). I will now have this dream, and fully recall and understand it upon awakening. I open myself to the highest possible insight and guidance." Then go to sleep, completely releasing the situation from your mind, resting in the expectation that you will receive the answer. As soon as you awaken write down your impressions.

Dreams are a level of consciousness that are not controlled by the conscious mind, and so can be an invaluable source of wisdom and guidance, free from bias. Many of my major decisions are based upon information I receive in the dream state, for I have learned to trust it as a reliable source that I can't color with my desires and expectations.

Natural Methods for Self-Healing

We do many things every day without even thinking about them that naturally help to restore our health. We may choose to wear a certain piece of jewelry, because we need the healing properties of its stone. On other days we don't feel like wearing it at all, the real reason being that our system doesn't need it.

Or we pick out a certain outfit that seems to complement us very well. On other days we might discover that we just don't look right in that outfit, because our energy field no longer needs the color for balance.

Or we crave particular foods at various times, and usually it is our bodies telling us that we need the vitamins or minerals they contain. Diet, incidentally, is an individual concern. You have heard that what is one man's meat is another man's poison. Each system is different, and our bodies will tell us what they need if we learn to listen. The truth of the best diet for you lies within your own being, and not in the current fad or austere program of self-denial.

What you eat isn't as important as how you eat, which should be in a relaxed manner. Sensitive people, especially those with low blood sugar, should eat four or five times a day, as I mentioned earlier.

Long fasts are not necessary because they deplete the body of vital reserves. Three day fasts occasionally are good cleansers, but these should not be strictly water fasts. They should be either juice fasts, or only eating things that are green on the outside (certain vegetables, watermelon).

At times you may feel especially drawn to taking long hot baths, which are excellent for relaxation. Or you may want to spend more time alone when your energy is down in order to rebuild it.

My channel has emphasized the natural healing forces all around us, and man's greatest natural gift for health and wholeness:

Nature is one of the biggest healers you have. Being outside in the sunlight feeds you, gives you energy, and helps restore balance. But even on a rainy or cloudy day the energy from rocks, trees, earth and water helps center and raise your energy field. If you have to work inside during the day you should surround yourself with as much greenery as possible, as this will provide you with extra energy.

Any form of creative expression is a natural healer. Dancing, playing or listening to music, painting, or whatever is using creative energy, will tap into the natural healing and balancing forces within you—as long as you are creating in a spirit of play and enjoyment.

Man's greatest natural gift for healing, however, is laughter. Laughter can heal all illness, and man would keep his energy high if he only kept his sense of humor. Then you could laugh at your mistakes and the mistakes of others instead of letting them get you down. The earth plane indeed provides a stage for all your dramas. Turn your suffering and tragedies into comical learning experiences, lighten up, and you will begin to know much greater joy and happiness. Don't you realize that God has a wonderful sense of humor?

Chapter 5

Sending Healing to Others

Group healing has great appeal because of its inherent power and support. You have probably heard the words from the Christian tradition: "Where two or more are gathered together in My name, there I will be, also." When people meet together in love, their combined energy field is much greater than the sum of its parts.

When someone is working with a healing group or another individual he experiences this heightened energy, love and caring. It often is just what he needs to awaken self-love and activate his own healing processes.

The best medical doctors are those who hold your hand, sending you love and energy. Often that is the most important ingredient determining whether you will get well.

Healing Is an Inside Job

We speak of healing others, but remember that healing is basically an inside job. When you "heal" someone you are really raising his energy level, activating the kundalini, and helping to create an environment in which his own healing processes take over.

A person can receive a jolt of healing energy, and appear to be cured for 48 hours. But after that time if he is not keeping his energy high, releasing the negativity that brought about the condition in the first place, the physical manifestation of the disease may begin to reappear.

Your Role in Sending Healing Energy

When you are participating in the healing process, remember that you are a pipe, a channel for the God energy. You might picture a sun of golden energy over your head, opening up and pouring through your being and out to the patient. Or you might imagine a shaft of light pouring into you and out through your hands. In this way you are linking up with the God source, and not pulling from your own energy field.

Remembering to do this has two important effects. First, if you give energy from your own field you will become depleted quickly, use up your reserves, and be subject to illness yourself. Second, by using the link up visualization you are reminded that all healing comes from God, and you can easily keep your ego out of the process. When one becomes emotionally involved or egotistically involved in whether a healing will occur, he gets uptight and begins to block the energy flow.

You must be relaxed to both send and take in healing energy. You might think of yourself as a straw, the energy just flowing through you. If you aren't relaxed you are like a flat straw, and nothing can get in or out.

You should always remain detached when sending healing, yet loving and compassionate. You should feel objectively removed. You are just a channel for the energy to flow through. You must not identify with the patient and pick up his aches, pains and negativity. Too many healers forget to detach themselves from the process, and wind up feeling the patient's symptoms. This does not help either you or the patient.

Remember that your only responsibility is to channel the energy and be as pure a vessel as possible. God's will takes over in the actual healing process. You don't have to be concerned about the result, for that is in God's hands! We do not help others by identifying with their pain. We help by providing extra energy for them to move beyond their pain and get insight into their condition.

When Healing Doesn't Work

Sometimes healings are instantaneous, sometimes they take hold over a period of time, but once in a while they may not seem to work at all. This does not mean your sincerity is lacking. It may mean that the individual receiving the energy is blocking it, failing to change his negative programs that brought on the imbalance. It may be that God is handling the situation in His own way.

Or there might be an imbalance between the patient and channel. To send the purest and strongest healing energy one should be in attunement with the patient. The greatest level of attunement is compassion and love. You learn to synchronize yourself as one, to communicate this oneness and wholeness to the patient so that he accepts this on some level of his being. This synchronization often takes a little practice. (You can picture yourself in your mind as an energy field, the patient as an energy field, and imagine that you are merging into one vibrant, dynamic, whole and balanced being. Sometimes this is communicated more readily to the patient through the use of your mental imagery.)

Can Everyone Heal?

If you care for others and want to give, it doesn't matter who you are or what you do. God uses all channels for healing. However, if your energy is low, if you are uptight, in poor health, you won't be as good a vessel for healing to flow through. This again is reason to remember that we must first love ourselves, take care of ourselves and keep our energy up if we would truly give to others. Because you can't give what you haven't got.

A person can send healing energy without really believing in it or understanding it. By practicing the healing techniques he can become an instrument of healing, even though he is ignorant of the process. When you open yourself to allow energy to flow through your body, your higher teachers can then work through you. My teachers have done many things that I didn't understand at all in the realm of healing, but I just went along and got good results. But the more you actually learn and understand about energy, the more you accelerate your own growth process, and the more effective healer you will be.

The most important single factor in sending or receiving healing, as I have emphasized, is that you be relaxed. When the body is not relaxed, the energy that is being channeled to you or through you will be blocked, and its effects will be greatly lessened.

You will also find that you limit your healing ability if you have a basic negative belief about it. When you open yourself completely, realizing that in God's power all things are possible, you become a much stronger channel. Also, you convey this faith to the conscious or subconscious mind of the patient. If the patient is initially skeptical, your faith in the process will help him relax and be more receptive.

The Basic Healing Group

For healing to be accelerated through a group, members and patients should meet at least once a week for a recharge. If the patient is doing his daily meditation, and there are no extenuating karmic circumstances (such as, the person has decided it is time to go home and the disease is the method he has chosen) he will get healthier and healthier, the rate of improvement depending upon his own free will and thought processes. When a person is sensitive and open it is easier to bring about a healing in a shorter period of time.

As I mentioned earlier, the group does not have to decide whether it is a person's time to go, and they do not even have to know what is wrong with him. Healing in its highest form is an outpouring of love, and in most cases the healing is allowed. The illness will not return unless the person fails to maintain his new orientation, transforming the conditions that brought on the illness.

Whatever method of healing the group may decide to use, it is always best to begin with a 10 to 20 minute period of meditation. This calms and centers all the energies, and if there is a negative group member it will mellow him out. It is helpful to have the patients meditate with the group when possible, as this will aid in relaxation, receptivity, and heightened energy.

Etheric Surgery

The basic technique used in ILF healing groups is etheric surgery. This was one of the first techniques given to me by my channel, and I have used it effectively for a number of years. But whatever healing technique you

Etheric Surgery

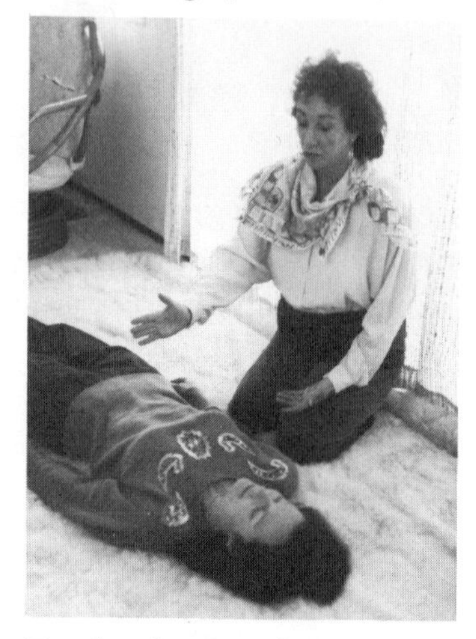

Turn hand on its side to raise person's kundalini. Move from root to crown chakra (see step 3).

Use up and down pulling motion with hand to perform surgery (see step 6).

use, you will never need to send energy for more than one to three minutes to a patient.

The basic idea of the technique is that you are working on the energy field, the etheric body, which corresponds to the physical body, and are correcting imbalances in the field. Everything is done on an energy level, so there is no need to physically touch the patient at all. The process involves the patient relaxing, lifting out the etheric body, doing surgery on the etheric body, and putting it back in the physical.

The steps are as follows:

1. Group members meditate for 10–20 minutes, preferably with the patient(s).

2. The patient lies down and completely relaxes. One group member sits at his head, another at his feet, lightly touching the patient. This sets up a polarity of energies. One member sits on the left side of the patient

to do the etheric surgery, and the other members sit on each side of the patient or in a circle around him, palms turned up. All members should imagine their link-up with the God energy.

3. The healer (person doing the etheric surgery) positions his right hand about six inches above the root chakra area of the patient, turns the hand straight out on its side, then moves it straight up toward the crown. (He is pulling up the patient's kundalini.)

4. Flattening his hand, so as not to lower the energy, he moves it back toward the root chakra, then straight out on its side again and pulls the energy up toward the crown chakra. He repeats this process five or six times, always keeping the hand about six inches above the physical body.

5. Next the healer moves his hand to the solar plexus area. (It is usually easiest to lift someone out of the body from this chakra.) Using the straightened side of the right hand again, and imagining it as a fish hook, he pulls up on the energy field and lifts the etheric body out about two or three inches. (Often people can feel the etheric body, and can feel the density when they begin pulling it up from the solar plexus. If you are unable to feel it, simply imagine it coming up and out and continue with the process.)

6. Let your hand move over the extended energy body and go to whatever area it feels drawn. Relax and go with what you feel. It will seem like your hand has an intelligence of its own, which is your teachers working through you. It will probably stop over one or two areas, and at these places you should begin an up and down pulling motion with your hand. The side of your hand is emitting energy which is cutting through the entire energy system. The hand should be straight.

7. After two or three minutes, bring the first three fingers of your right hand to your third eye, then point

the fingers toward the area you've been working on. You'll feel energy, like a laser beam, pouring forth from your finger tips. This acts as an antibiotic to the area the surgery was performed on. Then bring your hand up to your solar plexus where another source of energy is gathered. Then hold your right hand flat about 10 inches above the patient's solar plexus and slowly lower him back into the body. This you do as you lower your hand toward his solar plexus. Do not physically touch the patient, but stop two or three inches above him.

8. Sit quietly for another two or three minutes, relaxing in the energy and allowing the patient time to feel the intensified effects of the energy in his body. Surround yourself and the patient in white light energy.

The group members will probably feel a tingling in their hands, which is the kundalini flowing through them. And the patient will probably feel the energy from the etheric surgery all the way through his physical body. It's almost like electricity.

If the healer feels drawn to hold his hand still and channel energy into a particular area, he should flow with that. Each person is different, and the healer's intuition will be receptive to the individual's need, which will hasten the healing process.

If the patient or group members feel a little dizzy, it is the result of a great amount of energy flowing through them. They should then close their palms and give the energy a chance to balance out before continuing with the next patient.

Clearing the Chakras

Etheric surgery can be used in a one to one situation to cleanse each chakra and remove blocks. In this technique both the patient and healer are working together through visualization, and it has wonderful rejuvenating effects on each person. The two work as one unit, and often the healer experiences the same release and energy charge as the patient. This aids in the overall balancing of the system. The following technique uses the heart chakra as an example, but the same process should be used on each of the seven.

1. The patient sits down and relaxes, spine erect, and the healer stands to the side of the patient, right hand about six inches away from the heart chakra, left hand about six inches away from the corresponding area of the back.

2. The healer visualizes (and generally feels) an energy link between his hands, flowing through the heart chakra. The patient visualizes a disc of light in his heart center, about six inches in diameter.

3. The healer begins and continues the etheric surgery with the right hand for about one minute (holding the left hand still), using the same pulling in and out motion described in the etheric surgery technique above, as if pulling out all obstructions and blocks.

4. The patient relaxes and focuses his awareness on the disc of light in the heart center, imagining it growing brighter and brighter.

5. Then both take a deep breath, and as they exhale in unison the patient imagines the disc of light blasting out the front and back of his heart chakra, cleansing away all blocks and obstructions; and the healer pulls outward with both hands, away from the body about 18 inches, visualizing a stream of energy flooding out in each direction.

6. Then both sit quietly for a few moments, experiencing the increased energy in their beings.

Finding Energy Blocks in the Spine

You can learn to sense the energy blocks in the spine of another person simply by using your hand. Hold the right hand about six inches away from the spine, and slowly run it up and down from the crown to the root chakra. Wherever there is a block or tension you will feel a hot spot, or energy density. It is the energy of your hand responding to the energy field of the person.

I have done this many times and can always find the problem areas.

Although you cannot use your own hand on yourself, because you can't disassociate with your own energy field, you can learn to sense the energy blocks by tuning into your body through relaxation. As you begin

Finding Energy Blocks in the Spine

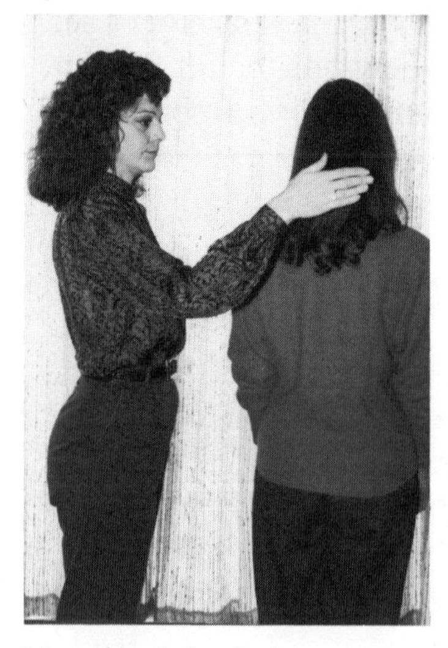

Move hand slowly from crown to root chakra to locate hot spots (hand about 6 inches from body).

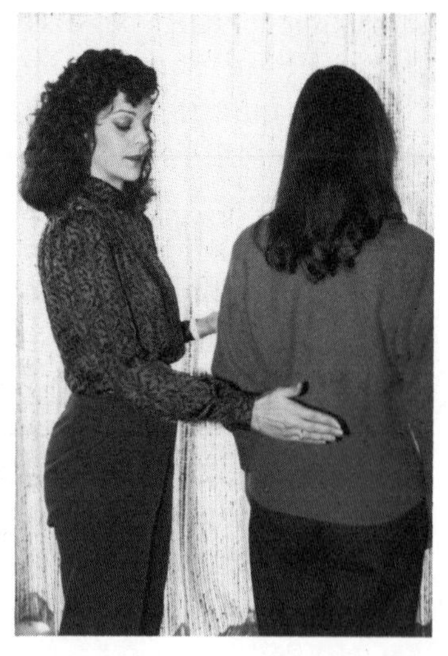

Continue same motion. Hold your left hand, palm up, to receive energy.

to relax, you will feel the tightness and perhaps some pain in these areas. Then you can use a visualization of energy flowing smoothly up and down your spine, seeing all the tension melting away.

The more completely we learn to relax, and the more we meditate, the more sensitive we become to our bodies and the easier it is to direct energy within to correct imbalances.

Burns and Cuts

If someone burns or cuts himself, you can use the etheric surgery over the area to help stop pain and hasten the healing. If used immediately there should be no scar

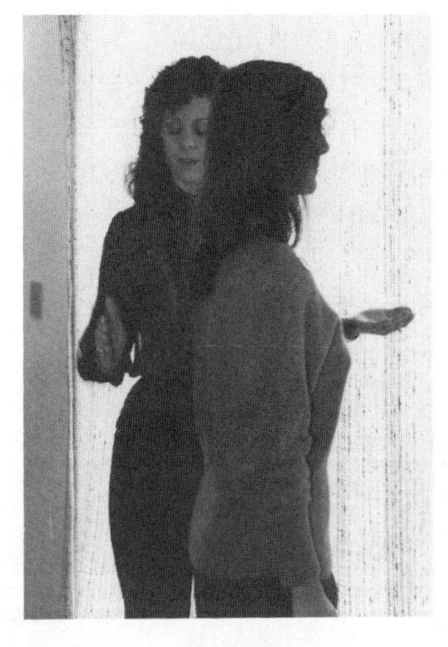

Stop when you feel a hot spot.

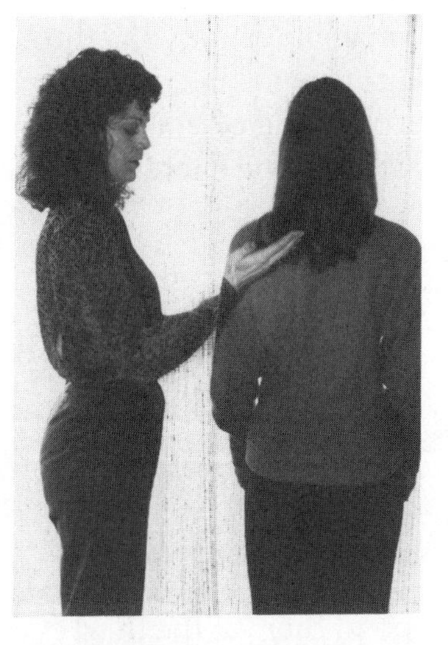

Use up and down pulling motion to break up energy blocks.

after the healing. You can also use the etheric surgery on yourself for such emergencies, for it works with the same beneficial results. Always apologize to your body and tell it you love it.

Laying On of Hands

The technique I use which most resembles the laying on of hands involves sending energy up and down the spine of the patient, activating his own kundalini. Stand behind the person, and place your hands on his shoulders. You might massage the shoulders gently for just a minute or two, to help the patient relax. Place your thumbs on each side of the spinal column on the back of the neck, and rest your fingers on the side of the collar bone.

Take a quick, deep breath, and then breathe out, linking up to the sun of energy over your head and imagining it flowing through your arms and hands, moving up and down the spine of the patient. (Energy comes out of your hands only as you are exhaling.) You are sending energy into the body, and the body knows just where to use it and what to do with it.

Sending Energy to the Third Eye

You can send energy to any chakra, and it will be utilized effectively in the body. The third eye is an easy one to work with, and is also good for eliminating headaches.

Using the first three fingers on your right hand, point them at the third eye area of the patient, either almost touching or touching the forehead. Imagine your link with the God source. Inhale deeply, and then exhale,

Laying on of Hands

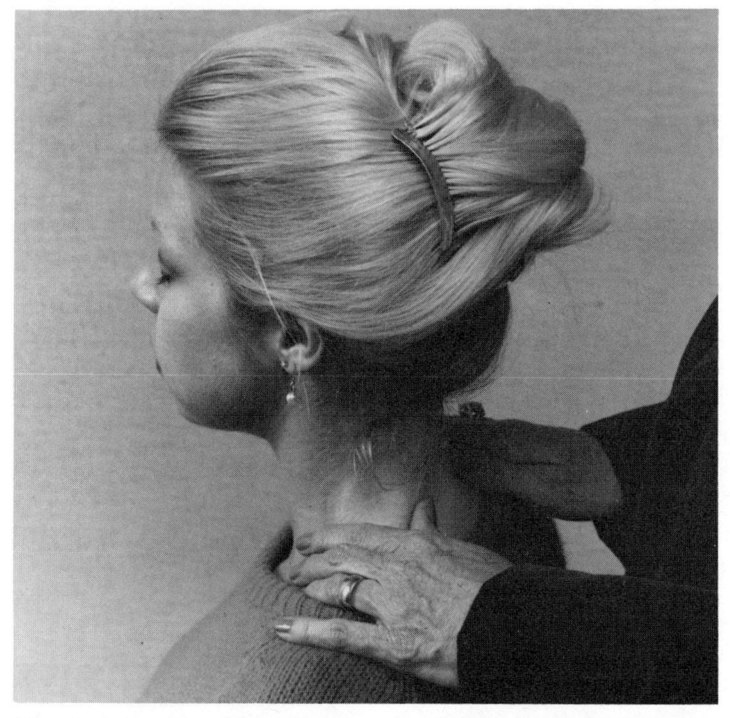

Place hands on shoulders, thumbs on each side of spinal column, fingers on side of collar bone.

imagining the energy flowing out through your arms and hands, flooding into the body of the patient. This is a great technique for giving someone an instant energy charge, in addition to disseminating the healing energy throughout the system.

Combing the Aura

This technique is designed to filter out impurities in the aura, to help smooth and balance the energy field.

Sending Energy to the Third Eye

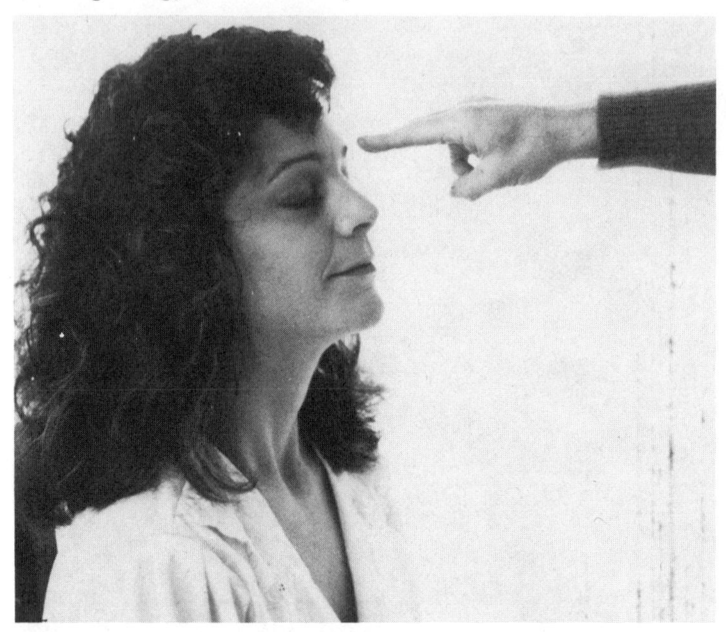

Use first three fingers of right hand, point at third eye area, not touching person.

The patient should be standing in an area large enough for you to walk around him in a circle of about eight feet in diameter.

Spread your fingers apart like the teeth on a comb, and, standing about four feet away from the patient, imagine that he is surrounded in an aura of white light. (If you visualize his aura it will be easier to comb.) Starting at the top of his extended energy field, reach your hands up, and pull them down to the feet. Continue to do this walking all around his energy field. By spreading the fingers you are not lowering his energy, but filtering it.

The patient will probably be able to feel the combing as a pleasant sensation in his physical body.

Fluffing the Aura

This is a fun technique that has an uplifting effect on one's spirits, and is especially good to use right after combing the aura.

Imagine a big fluffy cloud completely engulfing the patient, who may be standing or sitting. You walk all around him fluffing up the cloud's edges with your hands cupped. This fluffing motion uplifts the energy, and usually gets a chuckle or two from both the fluff*ee* and the fluff*er.*

Foot Massage

A good foot massage stimulates all the reflex points and energy systems of the body, and has a marvelous rejuvenating effect on you. There are points on the feet that correspond to every area and organ of the body, and by stimulating these points you can help restore balance

Fluffing the Aura

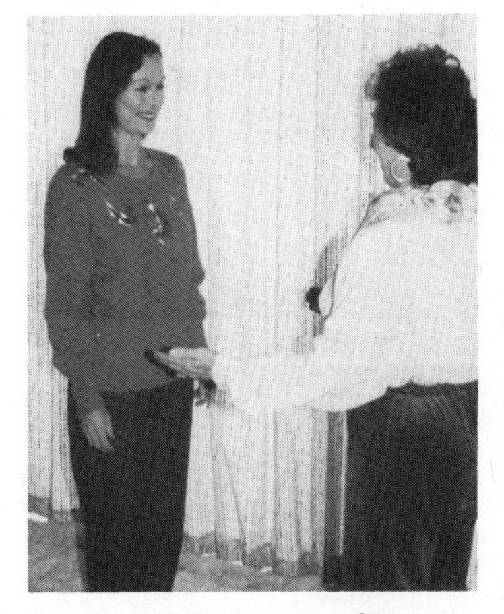

Cup hands for best results. Move from foot to head.

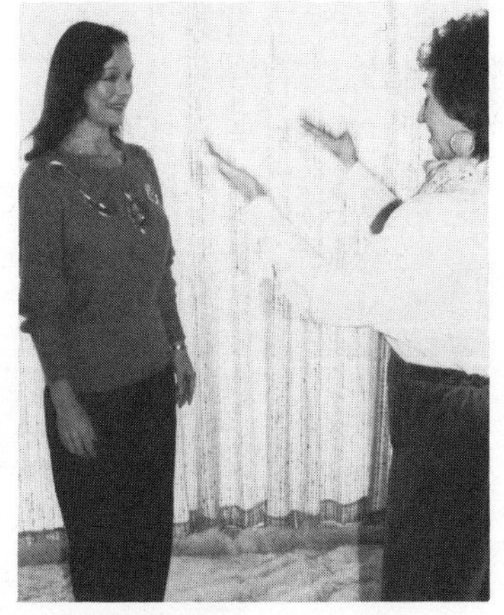

Use fluffing motion to uplift energy, walking completely around person.

and harmony. This system is known as reflexology. (See foot chart below.)

Although you may work with the specific points, it is not necessary to know them to give an effective foot massage.

Begin with either foot, massaging it gently with the palms of your hands, using a light oil if you prefer. Imagine that the foot is a piece of dough, and you are kneeding it, warming it up. Feet are often quite sensitive to pain, so be gentle as you go. Work with the foot about five minutes. Then press harder with your knuckles on the bottom of the foot, stimulating the entire area. If you feel little hard spots gently massage them. Work with

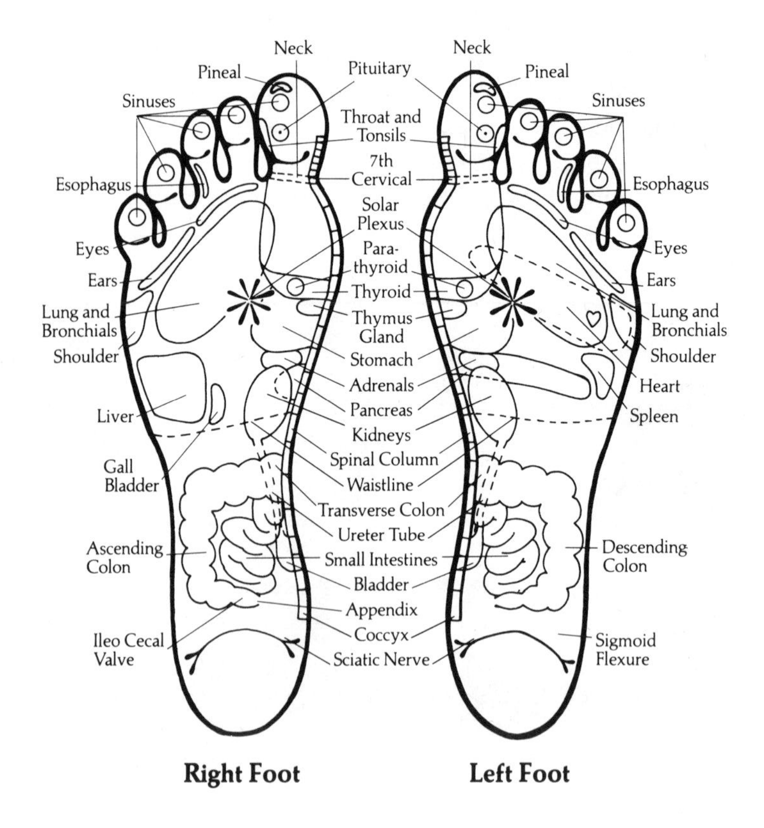

each foot a total of about 10 minutes. When you finish, the person who has just received the massage will feel like he's walking on air.

(Of course an all over body massage is a wonderful rejuvenator, too, but one needs to understand more about the muscle groups and energy centers to give a complete one. Just remember never to massage down, from the neck toward the base of the spine, because you will lower the person's energy.)

Absent Healing

You can send healing to others simply by visualizing them in a state of health and wholeness. Relax yourself completely, or begin the visualization before closing down at the end of meditation. Picture the person or persons in your mind to whom you wish to send healing. See them as happy, healthy, and engaged in some activity that suggests health and well-being. Concentrate on this image until it feels real to you, and create a sense of well-being within yourself, projecting it into the image. You might also imagine the persons surrounded in the white light of love and healing energy. Hold the image for one to two minutes, then release it from your mind.

Since time and space are no obstacles to sending healing, the persons have received the energy. They are free, of course, to accept or reject it, but since our natural tendency is toward health and wholeness, most people will not consciously or subconsciously block it (unless they have something invested in continuing to be sick: they like the attention, use it as an excuse to escape responsibility, or whatever).

The extra bonus is that whenever you send healing energy to another, or positive thoughts of any kind, you are also sending them to yourself. The blueprint begins in your mind, and the force of healing becomes active within your own being as well. (The other side of this, of course, is that whenever you send negative thoughts to another they also have their first and most immediate effect in your own system. That is why we cannot hurt or think negatively about another without also hurting ourselves. The Golden Rule captures this truth, for as we do and think unto others we are doing and thinking unto ourselves!)

Natural Group Healing

There are many forms of group healing we participate in every day. Some people are natural huggers. They love to hug and touch because this is their way of expressing caring to others. They have a lot of energy to give, and so they spread it around.

When persons are hurt or crying, we naturally reach out to hold them or hug them. This is giving them energy, helping them to gain a clearer perspective.

Smiles are great transporters of healing energy. When someone smiles at us from the heart, our whole day lights up. Smiles can communicate much love from a pure level of caring about our fellow man.

What you do in love, whether cooking, singing, writing, or any other activity, results in putting the love vibrations into it. This love will be felt by others who eat your food, listen to your song, read your book. Remember when we love we are healing, balancing, not only ourselves, but all with whom we come into contact.

Your high energy field is a natural healing device for others, for they feel uplifted in your presence.

In fact, everything we are, and everything we do, contributes to the building of harmony or disharmony, love or fear. In your daily meditation you are sending out healing vibrations through your own being, to your home, your community, even your world. And so we realize as we heal ourselves we are helping to heal others, and in the best sense we all become our brother's keeper.

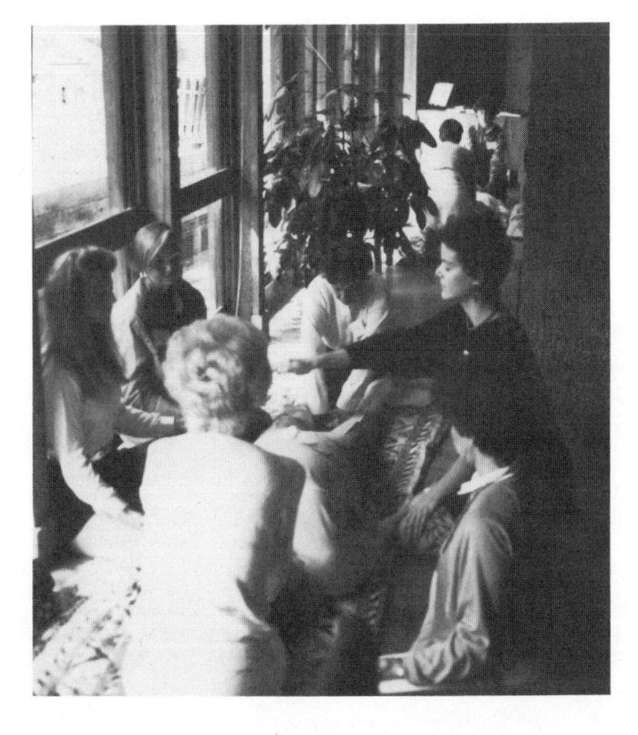

Chapter 6

Healing the World Through Spiritual Awareness

(A Trance Message Channeled by Betty Bethards)

Love Is the Secret

Basically all diseases are brought about through lack of spiritual awareness. True spiritual healing flows from the heart chakra, the Christ Center, and is the voice of love. Love is the secret of true healing.

Although it is true you can channel energy without really understanding the principles of healing, lasting healing must occur on a spiritual level, and that is the level of love.

At present mankind seeks to control the world through fear: fear of other nations, fear of power, fear of defeat, fear of holocaust. But fear is the cause of all disease and disharmony, whether on a personal, national or world level. Fear is the ultimate lack of spiritual awareness.

Man must grow to realize that he can control the world and bring its forces into harmony only through the power of love.

Wouldn't it be beautiful if all people were taught from the cradle onward that love is all they ever need, that any problem that ever arises can be solved through love, whether in family, one to one relationships, cities, countries or world situations? You have no idea of the power which lies within each one of you.

Man must tap into his creativity to begin to use this love force, to realize that all answers lie within, that creative solutions can be found to all problems of hardship and suffering.

Healing the world involves much more than feeding the hungry and clothing the poor, for this is putting a bandaid on the symptom, not dealing with the cause. It involves, as all great teachers have said, changing the inner nature of man. To do this man must bring into alignment his physical, mental and spiritual energy. He must truly recognize his oneness with all life and with the God force.

Seeing the God-Self

To develop the ability to see the God-self in everyone is what we mean by love. To truly love is to pour forth the God energy that is centered within the heart chakra of all people. It is learning to see all people as energy beings who are incarnating into human form to learn their lessons, perceive their destiny and to do that which they have chosen, which is unknown to any other.

Learning to love is realizing that you cannot judge another and you cannot be hurt. Each is a being of light, growing and learning, making mistakes, getting up and moving on, and each has his own pathway to walk. It may not be your pathway, but you cannot judge another path. You know not the person's past karma, and why he is following a particular way.

Thus it is essential that you tune in only to the good, the God, the essence of the spiritual self. As you learn to perceive within each being the things that are beautiful, you will manifest the beautiful within yourself, also.

And if you send out love, embracing the true being within, you will get back nothing but love. Another may send out anger and hostility, but it is his way of saying, "I'm hurt. I'm unhappy with myself so I'm unhappy with the world." As you practice seeing the divine spark, your compassion helps that soul see what he is trying to do with his life, to catch a glimpse of the Self within.

You can learn much from watching other souls. You can learn how to do or not to do something, and save yourself a lot of time through trial and error. But it takes a certain level of awareness to be willing to learn in this way. Many are too stubborn and insist on making their own mistakes.

The Second Coming

Many people today are waiting for the second coming of Jesus to take over the world, save them from their problems and solve all their difficulties.

But individual awareness is what the real second coming is all about. The second coming talked about in the Bible is not the coming of Jesus Christ or any other guru. Jesus does not intend to reincarnate. It is, instead, the coming of love, the opening of the heart center. the Christ within man.

The second coming is man's recognition of the God within. One need not believe in God or Christ as such, but through opening the heart center, he is indeed in touch with the love spirit within himself, and therefore touches the love spirit, the inner being, of all men.

The Guru Lies Within

In man's futile effort to find this leader who would save him and protect him, you see the rise of cults. Cults, however, are diversions from the truth. They are restrictive, authoritarian, and prejudiced against those who are not their own members. They tend to glorify the egos of the persons involved, and in time lose any spiritual perspective they might have had when they started.

One of mankind's ultimate tests is to be able to love all people, to truly know that every man and woman is part of his family. Man must become free enough to stand alone, not identifying with any rigid interpretation of doctrine, following the inner teacher of love. Yet at the same time he should feel at one with all he meets, honoring and learning from every other being, because he acknowledges the God self within all life.

Mankind can no longer afford to live like sheep, die for the wrong causes, for someone else's fear. He cannot afford to follow cult leaders and look for an easy salvation through the efforts of others.

It is time for you to take control of your own lives, to be your own Guru, to make your own decisions, grounded in a firm awakening of the love energy. One can always ask for insight and learn from all his brothers, but he must also be brave enough to follow what he feels.

That is why it is crucial to keep enlightening your awareness through practicing meditation. Your perception should come from higher and higher levels, your love energy growing stronger, and your motives becoming purer.

It is fine to be drawn to people who have charisma, for this is nothing more than high energy. But instead of basking in their energy and thinking how wonderful they are, you should be inspired to awaken your own energy to a higher level. Learn what they have to teach you and move on. You are in a universe of equal beings, and each one can teach another.

Many religious philosophies and belief systems are trying to make the search for truth very difficult. But the truth is simple, and always has been. Every answer you ever need to know on any subject lies deep within yourself!

The key is to be still, go within, and bring forth the answers. Bring forth the curative energy for yourself, heal your physical, mental and spiritual being; then bring forth the curative energy to the world.

Your whole perspective changes when you bring your inner forces into harmony. The world appears and responds to you in a completely new way, because you are coming from a perspective of love, unity, harmony and truth. It is only the beings with this awareness, and those working to achieve this awareness, that will be able to help their fellows in the critical times ahead for mankind.

The world needs all the love energy and healing energy possible, and this is the responsibility of each and every individual incarnating on the earth plane.

Heighten your awareness, develop awareness of your God-self, to see within the heart of man, to see the pain man brings upon himself and his fellow beings. It is not through being evil, but through ignorance of his true nature. Sorrow, disease, war, poverty, broken relationships — all these experiences are teaching you to know yourself, to get in touch with your needs, to follow your inner direction and purpose.

A Basic Lesson in Unity

Mankind today is stumbling along in darkness. But there are a few rays of hope emerging. Movements toward synthesis and integration, in the healing arts, in world religions, in international relationships, are gaining momentum.

But at the same time nationalism and petty rivalries are thriving, many countries and groups are fighting among themselves, man is killing his fellow man, cheating his friends, disregarding the older members of society. But there is much growth in store. Far more people are turning to the light, looking for answers. They are tired of violence, wars and poverty, and are choosing to face things in a united way.

What the United States was all about in the first place—its spiritual purpose—was bringing about changes in a united way, a union of people coming forth in one voice saying, "We care."

When mankind truly learns to care once again about himself, his family, his neighbor, his community, his city, his nation, and his position on this planet in relationship to all fellow beings, only then will the radiating power of love begin to take over and transform his world, and suffering can be eliminated.

There are many planes and levels of existence, many lessons to learn, universes to understand. The earth plane lessons are simple and basic, but at the same time are some of the most difficult to grasp. And learning the basic principles of the unity of all life on the earth plane is essential before moving on to higher planes of being.

An Exercise in Awareness

On a clear night, go outside and look up at the stars. Think about the millions of stars, the millions of galaxies, and the millions of life forms and levels of vibration in the universe. Mankind is but one wave of existence, one frequency or vibration, manifesting on a tiny planet in a tiny solar system amidst the infinite heavens.

Reflect for a few moments how great is Life, how great is Love, how great is God. How great it is that the very force which permeates all planets, galaxies, fellow beings and the entire universe is the very love force within each and every one of you. The sheer magnitude of this power is inconceivable to the mind, but it can be known in your heart. Creating harmony and peace on one small planet seems like such a little thing when you consider the magnificence of the force you are working with!

It takes but one thing: the realization within each soul of this force, this power of love. Persons who cannot decide what to do with their lives, who are depressed, who feel that life is not worth living — if only they could realize that they have chosen to participate in a spendid age, helping their fellows come into a realization of God consciousness. If only they could realize that they live at a time when every person matters a great deal because of the power and influence each can have on another. Never before in the history of your planet have you had such global communication systems available, such a powerful media system developed, and the consciousness of so many at a level that is ready to hear the truth of their beings.

The Importance of Learning to Heal

Recognizing your healing power and learning to heal is of critical importance in the present age. Healing is a way to immediately see the effects of the love energy. It is a way to quickly learn that the power of love, the God force, is real.

As man releases his healing potential, opening to the flow within him, he begins to work in harmony with his fellow man and to revolutionize the world. As you heal you awaken more and more your true spiritual self, and you awaken the spiritual self of all those you touch.

In this age it is no longer good enough to say to your children, students and friends, "Do as I say, not as I do." You are known by your fruits. Your own being is testimony to your inner balance, your inner radiance. You can transform the world and bring spiritual peace into the earth plane vibrations only by transforming yourself . . . in thought, word and deed.

You have the choice to learn to love yourself, to bring harmony into your life, and to radiate this harmony to the world you live in. It is your challenge, your opportunity, and your ultimate responsibility.